THE FAT-LOSS PLAN

JOE WICKS
The Body Coach

First published 2017 by Bluebird
an imprint of Pan Macmillan
20 New Wharf Road, London N1 9RR
Associated companies throughout the world
www.panmacmillan.com

ISBN 978-1-5098-3607-9

Credits
Publisher: Carole Tonkinson
Senior Editor: Martha Burley
Editorial Assistant: Hockley Raven Spare
Design: Ami Smithson
Food Photography: Maja Smend
Fitness and Opener Photography: Glen Burrows
Food Styling: Bianca Nice and Sunil Vijayakar
Prop Styling: Lydia Brun

9 8 7 6 5 4 3 2 1

A CIP catalogue record for this book is available from the British Library.

Designed and Typeset by www.cabinlondon.co.uk

Visit www.panmacmillan.com to read more about all our books and to buy them.
You will also find features, author interviews and news of any author events, and you
can sign up for e-newsletters so that you're always first to hear about our new releases.

**Bluebird publish books bringing you the very latest in diet,
self-help and popular psychology, as well as parenting, career
and business, and memoir.**

**We make books for life in every sense: life-enhancing but also
lasting; the ones you will turn to again and again for inspiration.**

bluebird
books for life

Contents

1

Introduction

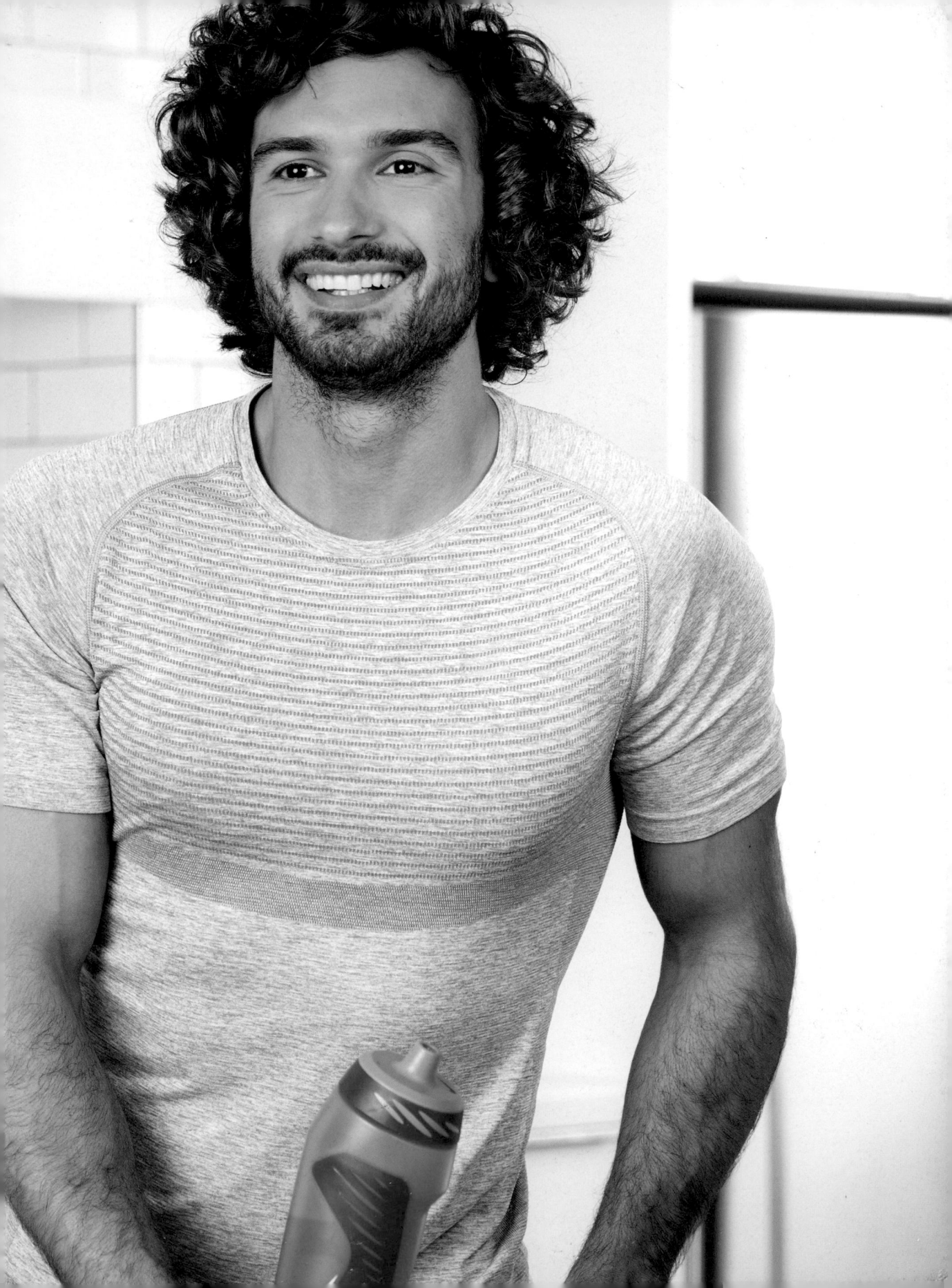

The Fat-Loss Plan

Hello and thank you for picking up *The Fat-Loss Plan*. The aim of this plan is to get your body burning unwanted fat and building lean muscle through a combination of food and exercise.

I truly believe that this book contains all of the information and tools you need to change your life and transform your body. I also believe that it's never too late to get lean and now is the time to start.

If you're fed up with counting calories or restrictive dieting, or you feel like you've tried everything before but failed, then this plan is for you. This is different. This will work.

My recipes are fast, my workouts are short and my philosophy is simple: stop dieting, stop counting calories, stay off the sad step, exercise regularly and cook real food.

You really don't need to go hungry, live a life without carbs or fats and spend hours on a treadmill to lose fat. That's the old way of doing things and it's not fun or sustainable. My way is much more enjoyable and a lot more fun.

My approach to food and fitness has already helped millions of people around the world get in shape, whether that's with my tailored online plan, my social media content or my cookbooks. I realised as soon as

I became a personal trainer that this is what I love doing the most – helping people overcome barriers and taking them on a journey to health, fitness and confidence.

I don't believe that anyone needs to be unfit or unhealthy and I know that the answer often comes back to good nutrition and exercise. This reduces the risk of illness, helps us to live longer, gives us energy and improves our self-confidence and happiness. This is why I want everyone in the world to stop making excuses, stop dieting and start living the Lean in 15 lifestyle.

I'm going to help you overcome the barrier of 'I don't have enough time' or 'I can't do it, I'll never be lean' once and for all. I'm going to inspire you to get in the kitchen cooking healthy food and to get up and start moving more.

This book is all about making lifestyle changes rather than a quick-fix solution. Consistency is the key to any successful fat-loss plan, and with my quick, tasty recipes and easy-to-follow home workouts, this book will fit into your life with ease.

It's going to take some commitment and effort on your part, but if you do commit to this plan, you will see your body fat melt away and you'll be more motivated than ever to keep going.

The recipes in this book are designed to make you feel awesome and energised all day, every day. I'll have you eating, fats, protein and carbohydrates to ensure you fuel your body correctly. There's nothing worse than a low-calorie, low-fat or zero-carb diet. That's not fun and it simply doesn't work. The body needs energy to burn fat and build lean muscle, so let's learn how to fuel it properly.

Ditch the calorie count

You'll notice that I don't list the calorie content of my recipes. This is for three very important reasons:

1 Counting calories is an old-school, outdated approach to nutrition. Not all calories are equal. For example, the body digests and metabolises energy from nuts, olives and avocados very differently to the energy given from biscuits, fried foods and fizzy drinks. This is why more than ever we need to stop counting calories and start taking it back to basics with real simple home cooking, which focuses on health.

We do need to be in a small calorie deficit to burn body fat, but it's way more important to focus on the quality of the foods and ingredients we eat and the way we prepare them over just focusing on the calorie content. My advice is to reduce your consumption of processed foods and focus on getting the majority of your energy from whole foods.

2 It's not realistic or healthy. Who wants to have to track, monitor and obsess over hitting a certain daily calorie intake? Not me. It's not realistic to think you can eat the same amount of calories or grams of fats, protein and carbs every day. I certainly don't count calories or track my macros. I just know if I eat three big healthy home-cooked meals, two snacks and do a good workout 4–5 days per week, I will stay lean all year round. I still enjoy meals out and the occasional night on the booze but I don't think about it too much.

Counting calories can also lead to unhealthy eating habits or eating disorders being formed. For example, 'saving' your calories to binge on unhealthy junk foods or massively under-eating and celebrating a super-low-calorie day of eating like it's a good thing. There's also the sense of guilt and disappointment people can have when eating out and not sticking to a certain calorie intake.

3 We are all totally unique individuals when it comes to nutrition. There is no magic daily calorie intake or macronutrient ratio. I think diets with a one-size-fits-all approach – for example, saying all men should eat 1400 calories and all women should eat 1200 calories – are completely flawed and inaccurate. This is because as individuals we all have different resting metabolic rates, body compositions, energy demands and hormonal balances which all affect our ability to burn fat. This is why you need to look at yourself as an individual and find out what it is that your body needs.

Perfect portions

I don't want you to think the portion sizes included here are perfect for your body, as they may not be. What I do want is for you to use my recipes for inspiration and, based on your own level of physical activity, adjust them accordingly. You may find the portions are too large for you or too small, so don't be afraid to listen to your body and try different things.

The quicker you learn how to fuel your body, the faster you will see results. You will digest food better, sleep better, recover faster, feel better and be more energised to smash your workouts.

A simple way to look at your body is as an engine. The food you put inside you – fats, protein and carbohydrates – is your fuel. You should only use the fuel that gets you revved up and performing at your best.

Good food gives you energy, and life is all about energy. I want you to know what I know about healthy food and how good it feels to just put goodness inside your body.

Winning motivation

I'm often asked how I stay motivated to exercise and eat well and my answer is always the same, 'I just want energy to feel good, be happy, be productive and to win at life every day.' Once you nail this, it's very easy to sustain a healthy diet and very difficult to go back to your old ways.

So here's to a new life full of energy, self-confidence and everyday happiness.

Good luck. Go and become the person who achieved their goal. This is your time to succeed. You can and will achieve a fit, lean and healthy body with this plan.

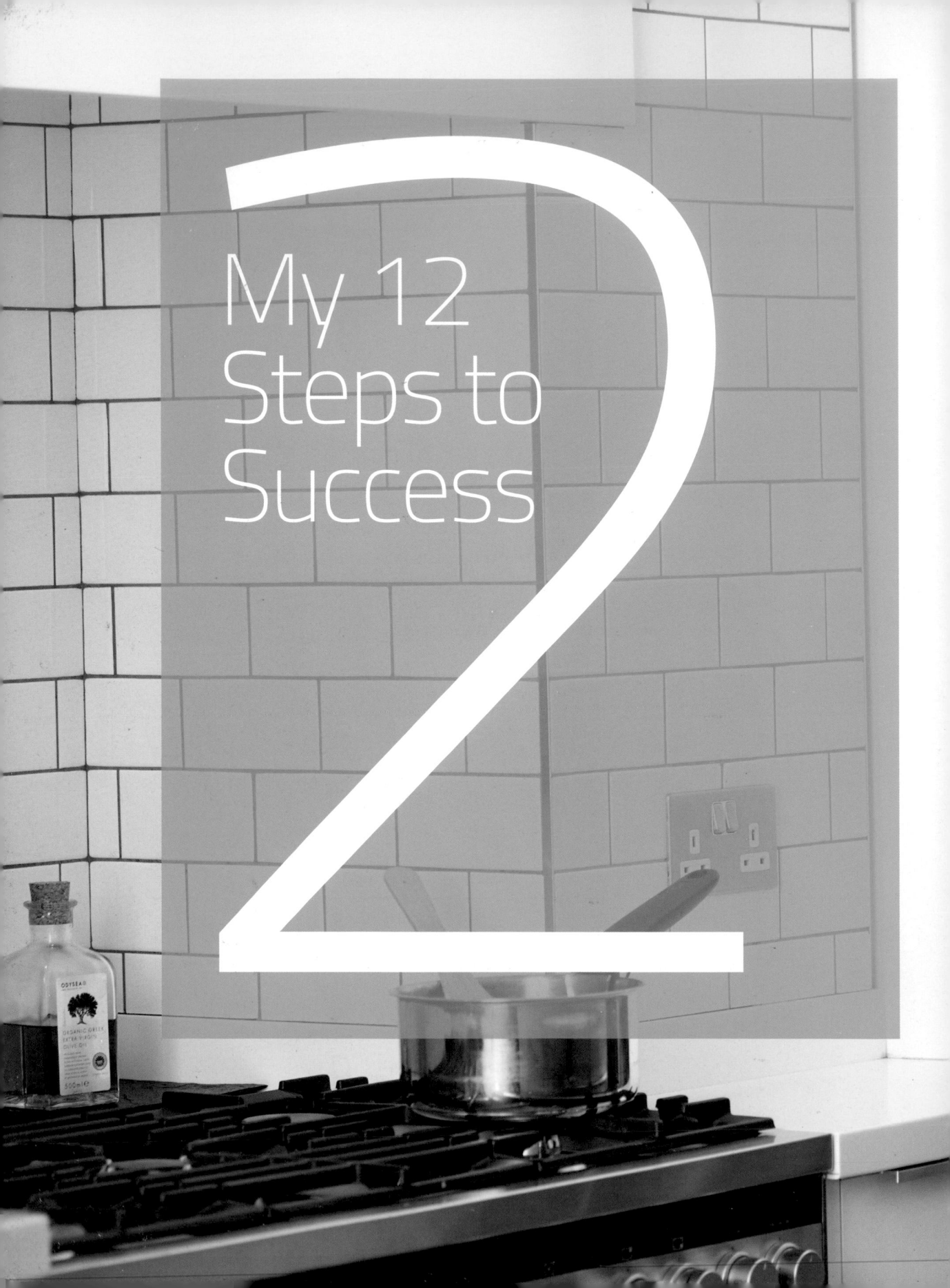

My 12
Steps to
Success

2

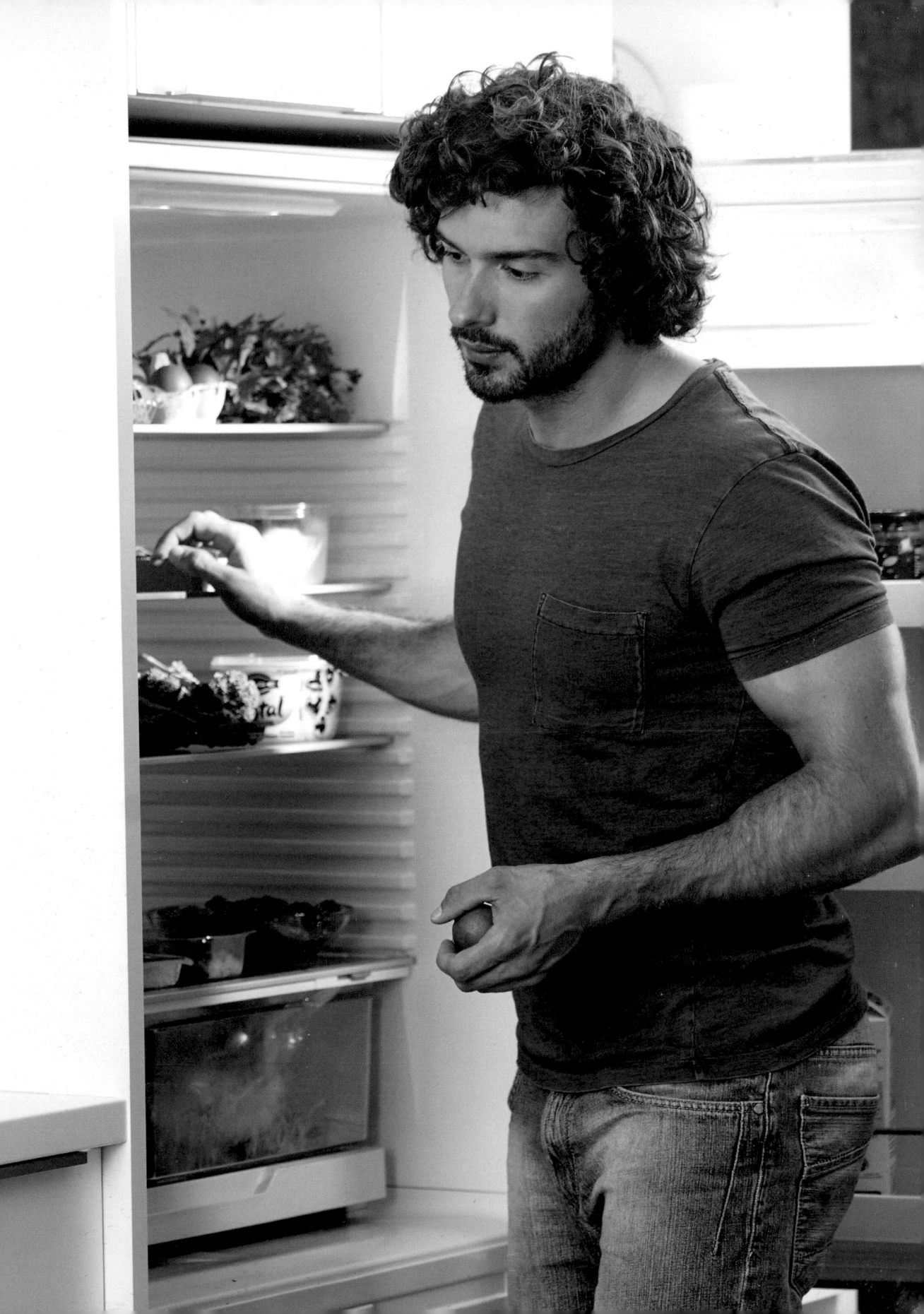

I have helped transform thousands of clients around the world with my online plan and I want *The Fat-Loss Plan* to be a success for you. This chapter includes the most important factors, behaviours and habits you need to form in order to sustain long-term fat-loss success.

Step 1: Throw away the sad step

I call the bathroom scales the sad step because ultimately that's what they are. The rapid weight-loss on the scales when you begin a new diet will motivate you, but only in the short term, as most of that initial loss will be water weight as opposed to actual body fat. This is often a result of an initial reduction of carbohydrates in your diet.

This occurs because the body stores carbohydrates in the liver and muscles as glycogen. Every 1g of stored glycogen is bound to 3–4g of water. This is why sometimes after a blow out or a heavy weekend eating carbs you can have silly weight gain on the scales like 6–10lbs. A lot of this weight therefore is water and not body fat, so it's very misleading.

Other factors affecting water retention are hormones and birth control medicine for women. During certain days in a menstrual cycle your body can hold more water. Being stressed can also increase a hormone called cortisol, which increases water retention, so again the sad step can be very inaccurate when measuring fat loss.

You'll stand on it and when the numbers don't move in the direction you want or as fast as you want it will make you feel sad.

It has the power to demotivate you and ruin your day in a single moment. The weight on the scales can therefore really

> **'The most motivating tool you can use is taking progress pictures'**

hide your true progress. It can leave you feeling like a failure. It can lead to you throwing in the towel or binging on food after your daily or weekly weigh-in.

The thing about the scales is they only measure your weight. They do not measure your body composition, your fitness or your confidence.

I've heard stories of people weighing themselves every single day. This is no way to live. So my advice is to throw the sad step out of the house. This may be a really big challenge if you are someone who has spent years weighing yourself, but it really is the first step to thinking differently about your body and feeling more confident and happy.

If you are someone who likes to measure stats, then use body circumference measurements such as chest, hips and waist to see real changes.

However, in my opinion, the most motivating tool you can use is taking progress pictures. Sometimes even looking in the mirror you can kid yourself into thinking you've made no progress, but photos can't lie. They show true changes over time. Take them at the end of each month from the side and front on. This will motivate you during the low points. The thought of taking a picture of yourself may seem scary but it's your chance to truly assess your body, set goals and wave goodbye to the old you.

Go on, you can do it. Throw away that sad step today.

Step 2: Stop counting calories

I touched on this in my introduction (see page 8) as it's something I feel really passionate about. This is the science: in order to burn stored body fat you need to be burning off more calories than you are consuming. This is defined as being in a calorie deficit.

> **'Life should be about enjoying your food and focusing on the energy it gives you. Not feeling guilty'**

When we consume more calories than we are expending we are in a calorie surplus. This is where we start to store excess energy as body fat.

Many fad diets out there focus solely on calorie intake without focusing on the quality or type of foods we eat. For example, you will be given a daily target of 1200 calories. This could then be obtained from anything from a meal replacement shake, low-fat yoghurt, a pizza, crisps or chocolate. Just because you are in a calorie deficit doesn't mean you are being healthy or happy for that reason.

I personally don't know how many calories per day I consume. It's very unrealistic to think that you will take in the same number of calories every day. You may eat at home one day meet your target of 1200 calories, then the following day you'll consume 2000 calories because you ate out in a restaurant or treated yourself to an ice cream. This really isn't the end of the world. It all balances out, and as long as you are in a small calorie deficit over the course of a week then you will still make progress.

It is, of course, important to be aware of the calorie content in certain foods, as even though something is healthy it doesn't mean you can eat unlimited amounts of it. For example, a handful of cashews (25–30g) makes a great snack but if you eat a whole 150g bag you could be consuming almost 800 calories in under 20 minutes. This could then put your body back into a calorie surplus and prevent you from burning body fat.

I think counting calories is an added pressure, which is totally unnecessary. It takes the enjoyment out of eating. Life should be about enjoying your food and focusing on the energy it gives you. Not feeling guilty about things or a failure if you don't hit a daily target.

My advice is to stop counting calories and start focusing on the foods you eat. Just by removing processed foods like sweets, fizzy drinks, ready meals, sauces, low-fat diet foods and replacing all these with recipes from this book you will naturally start to lose body fat. Then when you combine your new food choices with the workouts in this book you can say goodbye to unwanted body fat.

Step 3: Ditch the diets

If you're someone who has tried every fad diet known to man and has still not managed to achieve the body you want, this step is probably the most important one of all.

There are too many to even name, but you know the ones I'm talking about. The reason there are so many fad diets is because people by nature want instant results and rapid fat loss. This is often achieved by massively reducing your calorie intake, which isn't fun or sustainable.

If it is really as simple as just cutting calories and eating less than 1000 calories a day for a few weeks, everyone would be lean all-year-round. However, as you might have noticed from your own experience or that of your friends, when bodyweight drops rapidly, as soon as the diet ends and we return to a normal eating habits, we usually regain the weight lost and often add more on top.

This is because long-term low-calorie dieting actually decreases the body's metabolism through a down regulation of certain processes in the body and a loss of lean muscle tissue.

My belief is that you should never start a diet that you can't see yourself doing in a year's time. You need to enjoy your food and not obsess over certain food groups.

Cutting out carbs completely or banning all fats is also a very miserable way to live. This is where *The Fat-Loss Plan* is so effective, because nothing is banned. Nothing is a sin. I'm going to teach you to eat the right fuel at the right time to ensure your body burns fat for energy.

If you are a career dieter who has been on low-calorie diets and yo-yoed for years then it may seem counter-intuitive for me to tell you to eat more food, but that's what I am telling you. It is my biggest challenge to convince you to eat more as it's going against everything you've been told when it comes to dieting, but it's time to change your approach. The body needs energy to burn fat and build lean muscle. You cannot do this with a crash diet.

Step 4: Stay hydrated

Many people underestimate the importance of hydration and simply don't drink enough water. My top tip is to carry a one-litre refillable water bottle with you. Rather than waiting until you feel thirsty to drink, simply sip on it throughout the day. This is going to give you more energy, allow you to digest food better and will also help your body burn fat more efficiently.

From the moment you wake up, your number one priority should be to hydrate. After all, you have just usually spent 6–8 hours without any water. My recommendation is to drink 2–4 litres of water per day. By doing this you will be far less likely to crave snacks or drink empty calories from fizzy drinks, concentrated juices or alcohol.

It seems simple, but drinking more water really is essential for fat-loss. If you're a sweet drink addict and can't stand the taste of water, then try adding mint, cucumber, lemon or lime to your water bottle. It gives it a nice fresh flavour and will encourage you to drink more.

Step 5: Set yourself goals

If you're someone who struggles with motivation to stay on track with healthy eating and exercise, then this can really help you. I often write down small weekly goals to keep myself motivated.

Keep them simple and realistic. For example, you might schedule three workouts into your week: Monday, Wednesday and Friday. This is achievable and will make you feel awesome when you tick them off. The small daily wins all add up and enhance your sense of achievement and progress.

Goal setting is also important for fat-loss because with training progression comes results. Don't repeat the same workout every time at the same intensity. The body gets used to the same stimulus very quickly and won't change. By making things more challenging and aiming to break personal bests you will really give your body a reason to adapt, and this is when you break through plateaus and transform your body. You might set a goal to do two more reps or run 2mph faster on your next HIIT. These small incremental progressions are the difference between staying exactly the same and transforming your body.

Aim to beat yourself and improve week on week. It might be a good idea to keep a training diary to help you with goal setting.

Another long-term goal is to keep really positive for staying motivated. For example, aiming to fit into a special dress or suit for a New Year's Eve party, or signing up to a fitness challenge with a friend. It's these things in the diary that will keep you going when the winter months come and training becomes harder.

Step 6: Get a good night's sleep

This is another very important thing to consider for fat-loss. If you are someone who stays up late or gets a lot of broken sleep then this could be something holding your body back from burning fat.

On a really simple level, if you are really tired you will not have the energy to exercise. You probably won't even be bothered to try, and if you do it will be a half-hearted workout. And you certainly won't be in the mood to cook and prep meals either,

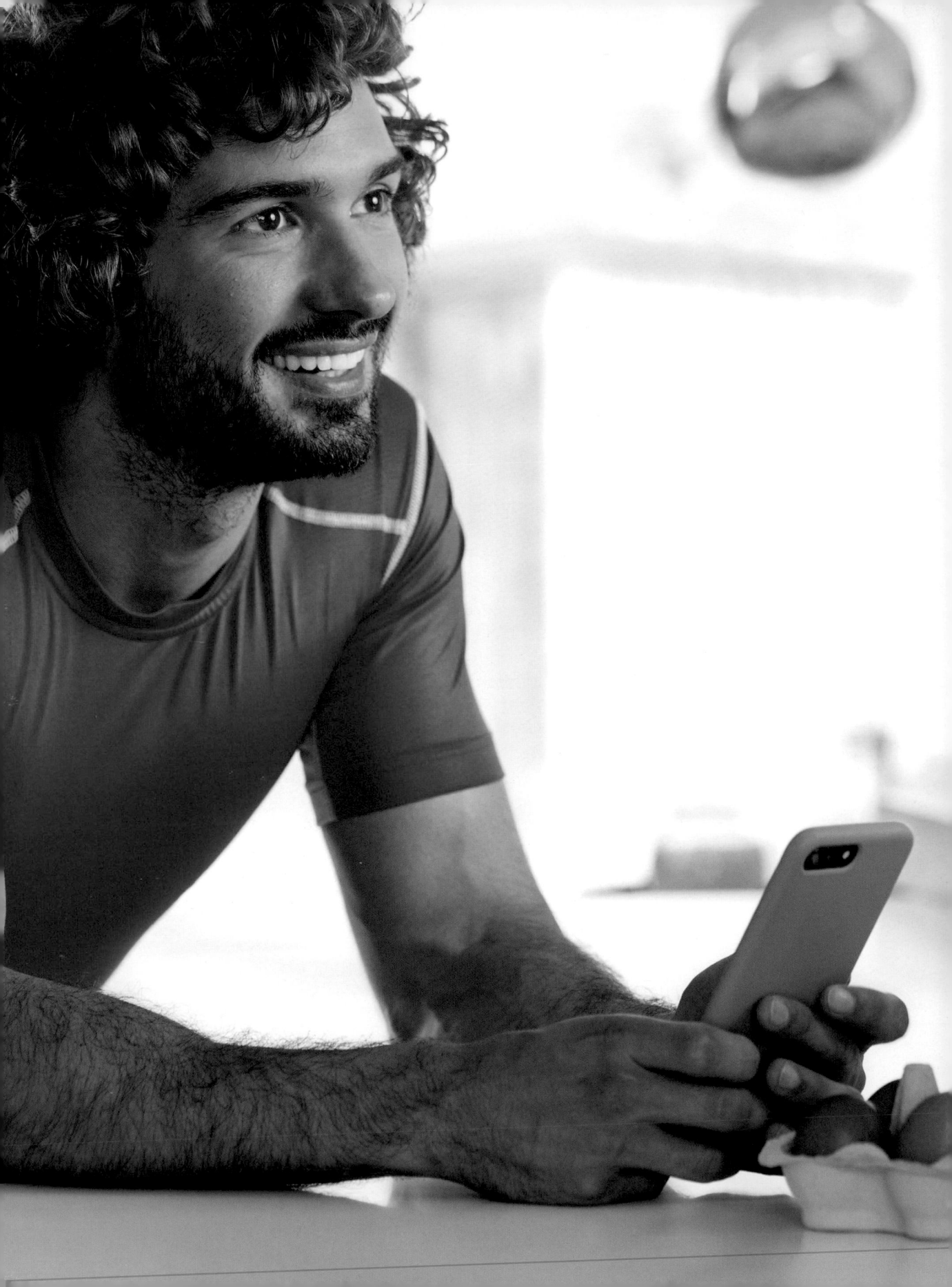

so being tired means you'll end up in a rush and more than likely end up buying convenience or junk food on the go.

Not only this but when the body is tired the brain starts to really crave carbohydrates, and these are often grabbed in the form of simple sugars in fizzy drinks, energy drinks, chocolates or sweets.

The simple practice of getting to bed an hour early and waking up to do a quick 25-minute workout is literally life changing.

You go from feeling tired to feeling energised. From feeling low to feeling buzzing. It's something I truly believe makes you a better person and allows you to get more done every day.

Because of my morning workouts I'm more patient, more focused, more productive and just nicer to be around. I'm happier every day when I exercise. I also make much better food choices if I'm eating out because I think, well, I've pushed my body through a really intense workout now so I deserve to show it some love with some healthy food.

When you start to see all these small steps in the bigger picture you realise that they are all as important as each other in a way, because one has a huge positive impact on the next.

A tired person doesn't function well. As clichéd as it sounds, just switch off your TV and phone an hour early. Listen to some nice music and nod off an hour earlier than you normally would. This will set up your day to a good start. It's giving you a chance to go and win the day.

Step 7: Throw away the bad stuff

I'm all for having a treat. I believe you should enjoy the food you love and celebrate with the occasional treat, but if you are someone who struggles with self-discipline and find yourself boshing a whole packet of chocolate Hobnobs before bed then this is so important for you.

If the sugar monster is stronger than your willpower then you need to remove the bad stuff from your life. These foods may seem like a treat because they taste good at the time but they are also the thing holding you back from getting lean and feeling fit and confident in your body.

To give yourself a real chance of actually burning body fat and seeing your body transform you need to take your shopping trolley, fridge and cupboards on their own transformation. By removing the fake food – chocolate, biscuits, crisps, cereal, low-fat yoghurts, sweets, ready-meals, bottled sauces and fizzy drinks – from your weekly shop you are making a big leap towards progress.

I often speak to parents who say this is really hard to do when you have young kids, but remember, you are the boss and you also want to make sure they grow up to be healthy so this is going to benefit them too in a big way.

By cutting out all this crap with refined sugars they will wake up with more energy, go to school and be more focused and more productive, so in all honesty you are literally going to help your kids become smarter.

Of course you're going to buy the odd treat now and again while out and about but you won't have it there in the house every night when your cravings come and the sugar monster comes to get you before bed. You are removing the temptations and increasing your chances of going home to cook real food – food that won't drag you down and make you feel crap but will elevate your energy levels and make you feel awesome.

Now you've removed the bad stuff, you can go and start filling your trolley with proper food: single-ingredient nutrient-dense stuff, such as nuts, fish, meat, fruit, vegetables, nuts, cheese, avocados, eggs, butter, oats, rice and potatoes.

Never go food shopping when you are starving hungry. I've done it myself before and it's insane how bad my food choices become when I'm walking around hungry. OMG my basket looks like a kids' party – half of which I eat on the way out of the supermarket and in the car before I get home! Bags of cookies, tubs of ice cream and cartons of orange juice all get in when usually I wouldn't even think of buying this sort of stuff. Have a healthy meal or snack before you go shopping and I'm confident you will not crave the junk foods you usually do.

Just a quick tip on BOOZE, too. I don't like to be the bearer of bad news but I want to lay it down on the line so it's completely clear to all the people who love a glass of wine or beer with their dinner. The simple fact is that the body cannot store alcohol. Therefore when you consume it, regardless of the type of spirit, beer or wine, the body must get rid of it. Yes, some drinks are higher in calories than others, but essentially by consuming alcohol in any form you are putting the brakes on fat burning. This means the less alcohol you consume the more body fat you will burn.

Step 8: Prep like a boss

I talk about this a lot on social media because the fact is prepping like a boss is the key to long-term sustained fat-loss. What I mean by this is learning to cook and prepare your own food. Being confident in the kitchen and taking control. Batch-cooking meals so you can carry your lunch to work or have dinner ready to go when you get in from a long day.

The busier and more hectic your lifestyle the more important this step becomes. If you work from home and don't have kids, the chances are you have it pretty sweet and can cook all meals from scratch. But if you have a busy house with kids or you work shifts then this is paramount for your success.

By planning your meals on a Sunday or during the week for the week ahead you are setting yourself up to succeed.

I am going to teach you how to batch-cook certain recipes so you can eat some for dinner and have some for lunch the following day. You can make breakfast the night before so after your morning workout you can shower and eat and get on your way much quicker.

This feels like a pain in the backside to begin with but it soon becomes a habit. It means you don't have to skip breakfast or eat some really sugary cereal before work. It means you will have more control over your nutrition and won't have to rely on food on the go all the time.

In the long run it will also save you money because nowadays eating out every day and buying a coffee soon adds up. By food shopping smarter and buying in bulk I believe you will be better off financially over the year.

Step 9: Don't go hangry

I think to an extent we are all emotional eaters. When we feel happy and in control we want to eat certain foods and when we feel sad, stressed or angry we choose to eat other stuff to make us feel better.

I'm hoping that by following steps 1–8 you will not experience this as much because you would have ditched the low-calorie diets, be eating more food and have cleared out the bad stuff you usually reach for.

Binging often occurs when people skip meals and go for long periods without food, or when they try to get through the day on low-calorie diets.

If like me you get hangry … don't go hungry. An emotional binge-eating session often feels like a great idea at the time

> **'Next time you feel like a blow-out, do something you never regret – a short workout'**

but you know that not long after you will start to feel down about it. You regret it. You wake up really tired or your tummy hurts.

Next time you feel like a blow-out, do something you never regret – a short workout. I can almost guarantee you will feel so much better and will make better food choices.

Step 10: Be patient, be consistent

The problem with most people is they want success and they want it right now. I'm so fed up with seeing books on losing 14lbs in 14 days and 7lbs in 7 days, promising quick fixes to get you in shape for your holiday. They don't mention the fact most of that sort of sudden weight-loss is water or that you will regain all the weight you've lost once you go back to eating like a normal human.

The reality is, fat-loss takes time. It's a journey not a race and needs to be gradually chipped away at. This refers back to step 1 (Throw away the sad step).

Unfortunately, the annoying thing about body fat is that it can be very, very stubborn. It comes on way quicker than it appears to come off and this is the problem. You need to think long term. Depending on where you are starting from you need to be realistic. It may take you 90 days to reach your goal, or it may take a year. This is where you need to be patient and be consistent.

Don't be disheartened if you know someone who is losing weight quicker or compare yourself to any other body. Your body is unique and we all burn body fat at different rates depending on various factors such as age, body composition, training intensity and hormones. As I said before, progress pictures will motivate you way more than just weighing yourself on the scales.

Accept that changes can be really annoyingly slow, but do not let this faze you. Let it motivate you to push harder, to mix up your training, to make small changes to your nutrition.

On days when you feel like you've hit a plateau, look back at old photos and remind yourself how far you have come. Don't let it get you down and cause you to go on another binge or to try another silly crash diet. More than ever, you now need to keep going, because if you let your impatience derail your efforts you will never reach your goal.

The only option you have is to keep moving forward. Keep prepping like a boss, keep training hard and stay consistent.

Step 11: Believe in yourself

This step is all about removing any limiting beliefs you have about your ability to succeed on this plan. You may have been dieting for 20 years or you may have never even tried to get lean in your life, but one thing you must retain throughout this journey is self-belief.

Success will not happen overnight. The body takes time to adapt to a new diet and results may be slower than you want. This does not mean you throw in the towel and revert back to your old methods. Remember, the dieting you've done hasn't worked in the past and it won't suddenly start working now.

Tell yourself you do have the ability to change your habits. You do have the power to say no to bad foods and the discipline to stick to this plan. When you believe in yourself and only focus on the positive changes you are making then you will achieve your goal. So don't even entertain the idea of failure, because this time is different. You are now going to become the person you want to be, because you can.

Step 12: Exercise and happiness

I'm not a neuroscientist or a psychologist but one thing I'm certain of is that exercise makes me feel good. If I wake up feeling a bit flat or low in my mood then I aim to do a 25-minute workout before anything. It takes willpower to get started but without fail I never regret a workout and always feel better afterwards.

I don't personally suffer from depression but I've worked with thousands of clients who do and they all agree that exercise is the best cure and the quickest way to feeling better. If you're someone who suffers from anxiety or depression or you just find you feel low on some days, then exercise really is the cure. It may feel like the last thing you want to do but if you can, just get going – even when you're exercising for 10–15 minutes your brain will release those wonderful endorphins.

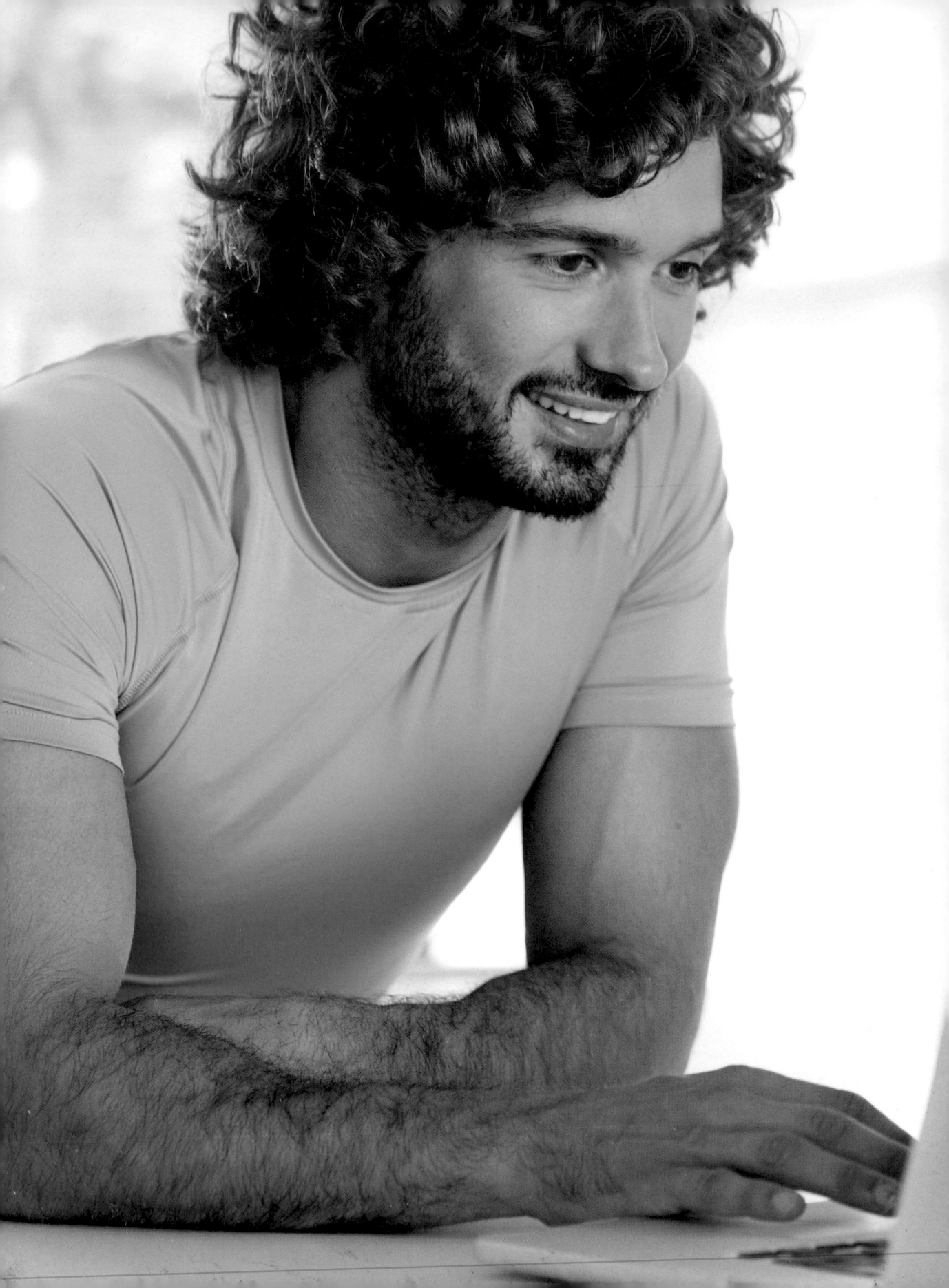

3

Getting
Started

The recipes in this book are divided into three sections: Reduced-carb, Post-workout and Snacks and Sweet Treats. Some of the sweet treats are a bit naughty so remember they are to be eaten occasionally but not every day.

I personally feel my body runs best when having one big carb meal and two reduced-carb meals on a training day, and recommend this below. If you find this also gives you loads of energy and makes you feel good then stick with that. If you feel better eating three carbohydrate-rich meals a day instead, then that's what you should do.

Reduced-carb meals

These meals are lower in carbohydrate than Post-workout meals, but higher in fat and protein. This doesn't mean the meals are low-calorie, though. We are just getting more energy here from fats instead, which have been shown to keep you feeling fuller for longer but also help maintain stable blood-sugar levels.

The recipes are all full of protein, high in fat, low in carbohydrate, without added sugar. Protein-rich portions here with eggs, nuts and cheeses and supplementing fats with avocados and coconut milk.

Post-workout meals

These are low in fat but high in protein and carbohydrate. This is just what the body loves to refuel so eat these meals after exercise.

These meals are high-carb, full of protein and contain much less fat than the Reduced-carb meals.

Opposite is a sample week of training and eating for me. I like to train 5 days per week with 2 full rest days. If this is totally unrealistic for you, simply plan your week accordingly, then choose your meals for the week ahead.

WORKOUT DAY

2 x Reduced-carb meals
1 x Post-workout meal
2 x Snacks

REST DAY

3 x Reduced-carb meals
2 x Snacks

	Monday	Tuesday	Wednesday	Thursday	Friday	Saturday	Sunday
	WORKOUT	WORKOUT	WORKOUT	REST	WORKOUT	WORKOUT	REST
BREAKFAST	Joe's Bounty Overnight Oats	Spinach and Goat's Cheese Omelette	Raspberry, Banana and Buttermilk Pancakes	Spicy Scrambled Eggs	Spring Onion, Bacon and Tomato Tortilla	Lean Green Smoothie	Turkish-style Eggs with Roasted Peppers and Yoghurt
SNACK 1	Cashew and Coconut Energy Balls	75g blueberries	Apple	Cashew and Coconut Energy Balls	30g nuts	Boiled egg	Joe's Little Balls of Energy
LUNCH	Thai Chicken Lettuce Wraps	Grilled Harissa Chicken and Chickpea Salad	Joe's Veggie Super Bowl	Beetroot, Feta and Chicken Salad	Sweet 'n' Sticky Chicken with Beans and Lentil Salad	Breakfast Ham and Chicken Club 'Sub'	Mango, Chicken and Avocado Salad
SNACK 2	30g nuts	Avocado Hummus with Super Seed Dukkah	Joe's Little Balls of Energy	75g blueberries	Apple	Avocado Hummus with Super Seed Dukkah	Apple
EVENING MEAL	Naked Lamb and Feta Burger with Beetroot Relish	Toasted Ciabatta with Fillet Steak and Harissa	Tandoori Chicken with Cauliflower Pilau Rice	Maple-glazed Lamb Chops with Creamy Kale	Prawn, Chilli and Tomato Linguini	Spicy Chipotle Chicken Bowl with Chunky Guacamole	Moroccan Salmon and Prawn Fish Cakes

Reduced-carb

Post-workout

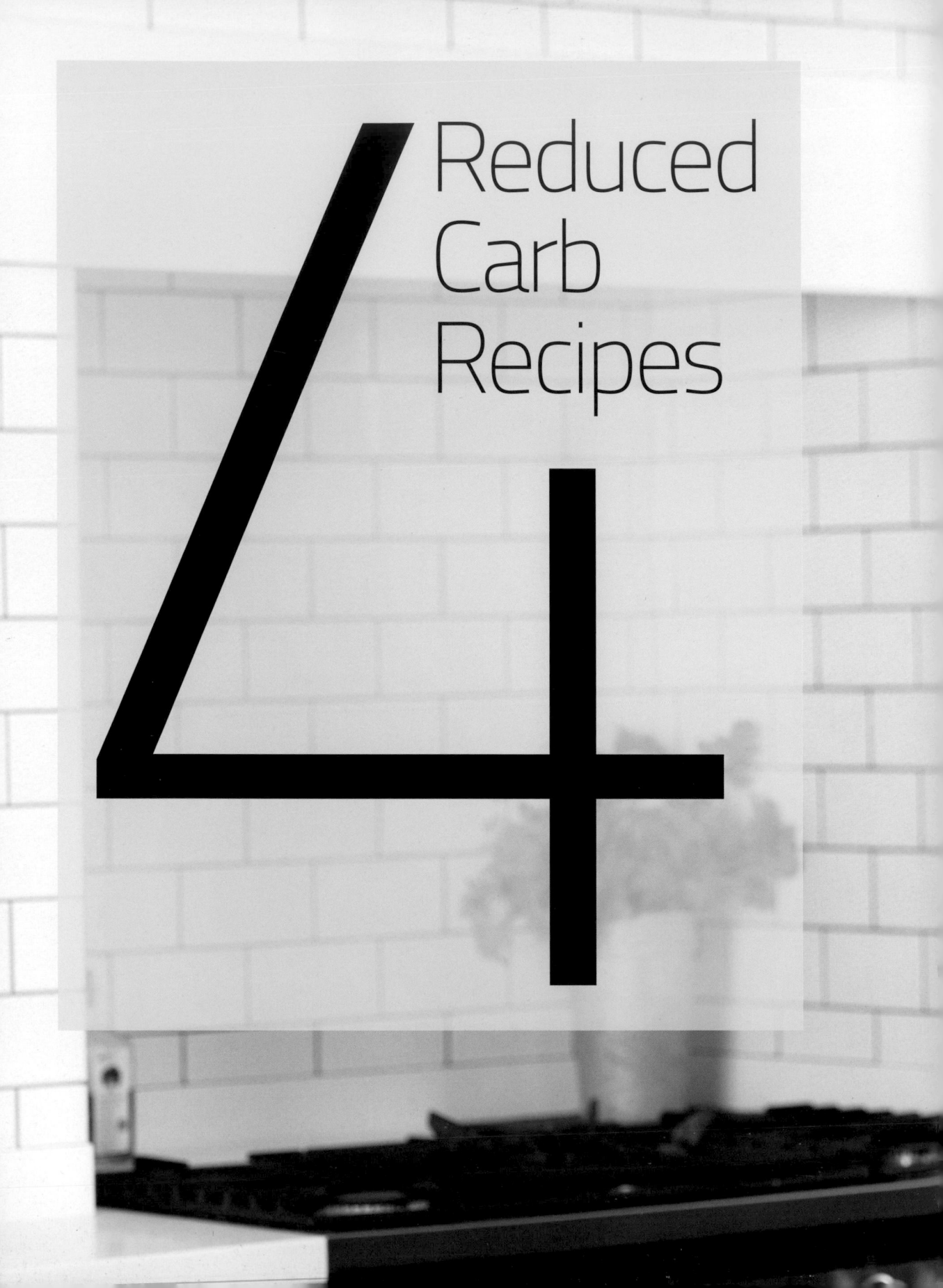

4

Reduced
Carb
Recipes

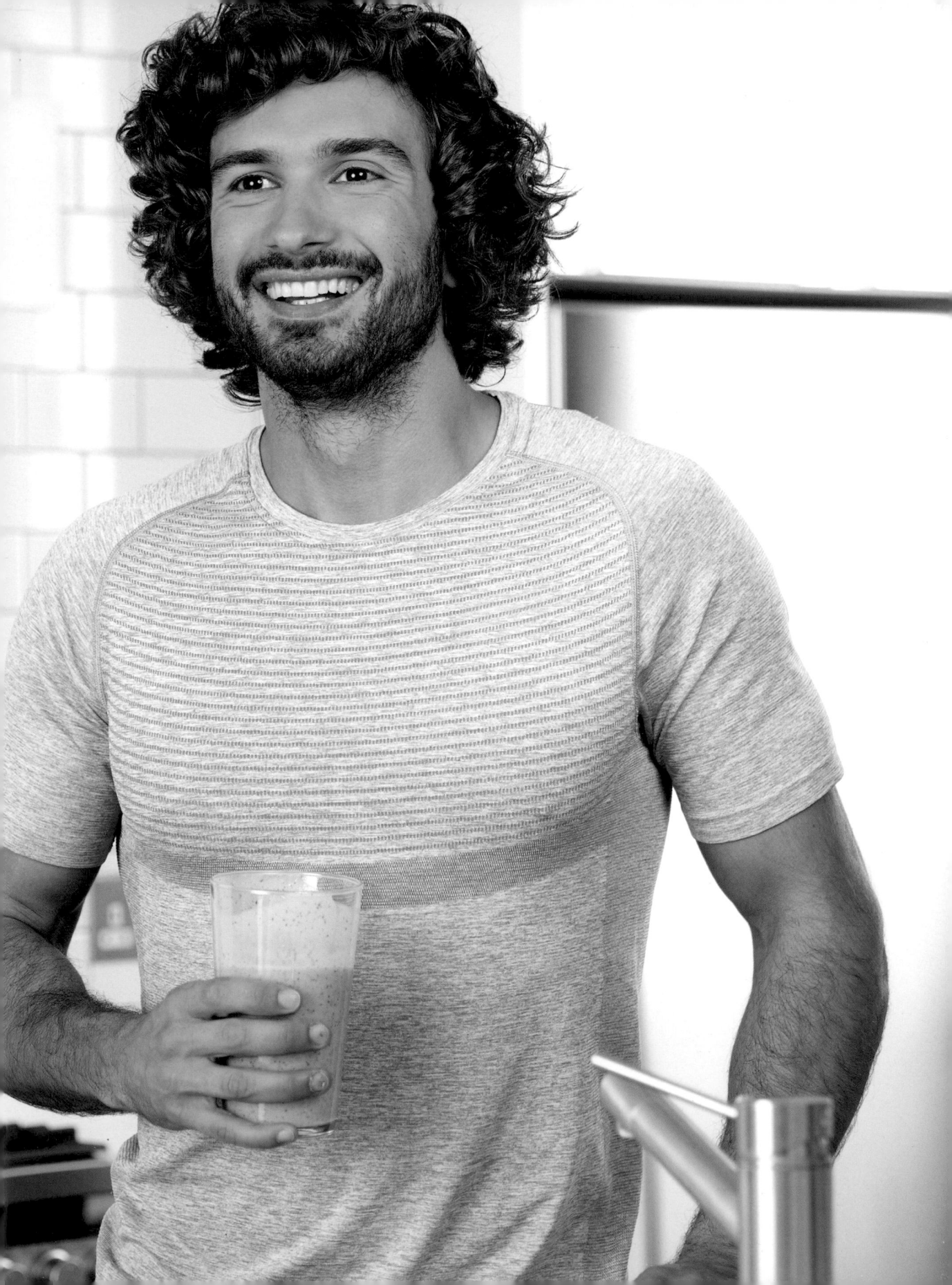

🕐 Make ahead

Lean Green Smoothie

This is a great grab-and-go option if you're rushing to leave the house in the morning. The fats in the avocado will provide you with plenty of energy and the greens are full of vitamins and antioxidants.

Ingredients

1 avocado
40g baby spinach leaves
1 tbsp mint leaves, chopped
200ml apple juice
100ml almond milk
1 scoop (30g) vanilla protein
   powder

Method

Halve the avocado and remove the stone. Scoop the flesh into a blender. Roughly chop the spinach and chuck it into the blender with the mint, apple juice, almond milk and protein powder.

Blitz until well combined and creamy. Pour into a tall, chilled glass and serve.

Serves
1

🕐 Make ahead

Mango and Passionfruit Smoothie

This tropical smoothie will brighten up any day of your week. This is another on-the-go option for work that tastes amazing.

Ingredients

100g frozen mango chunks
½ banana
60g coconut yoghurt
1 scoop (30g) vanilla protein
   powder
1 ripe passionfruit
1 tbsp chia seeds

Method

Place the mango, banana, coconut yoghurt and vanilla protein powder into a blender.

Scoop the passionfruit pulp into a sieve over the blender, reserving the seeds. Top up the blender with 250ml water and blend until smooth. Pour into a glass, stir through the passionfruit and chia seeds and drink it down.

Reduced-carb

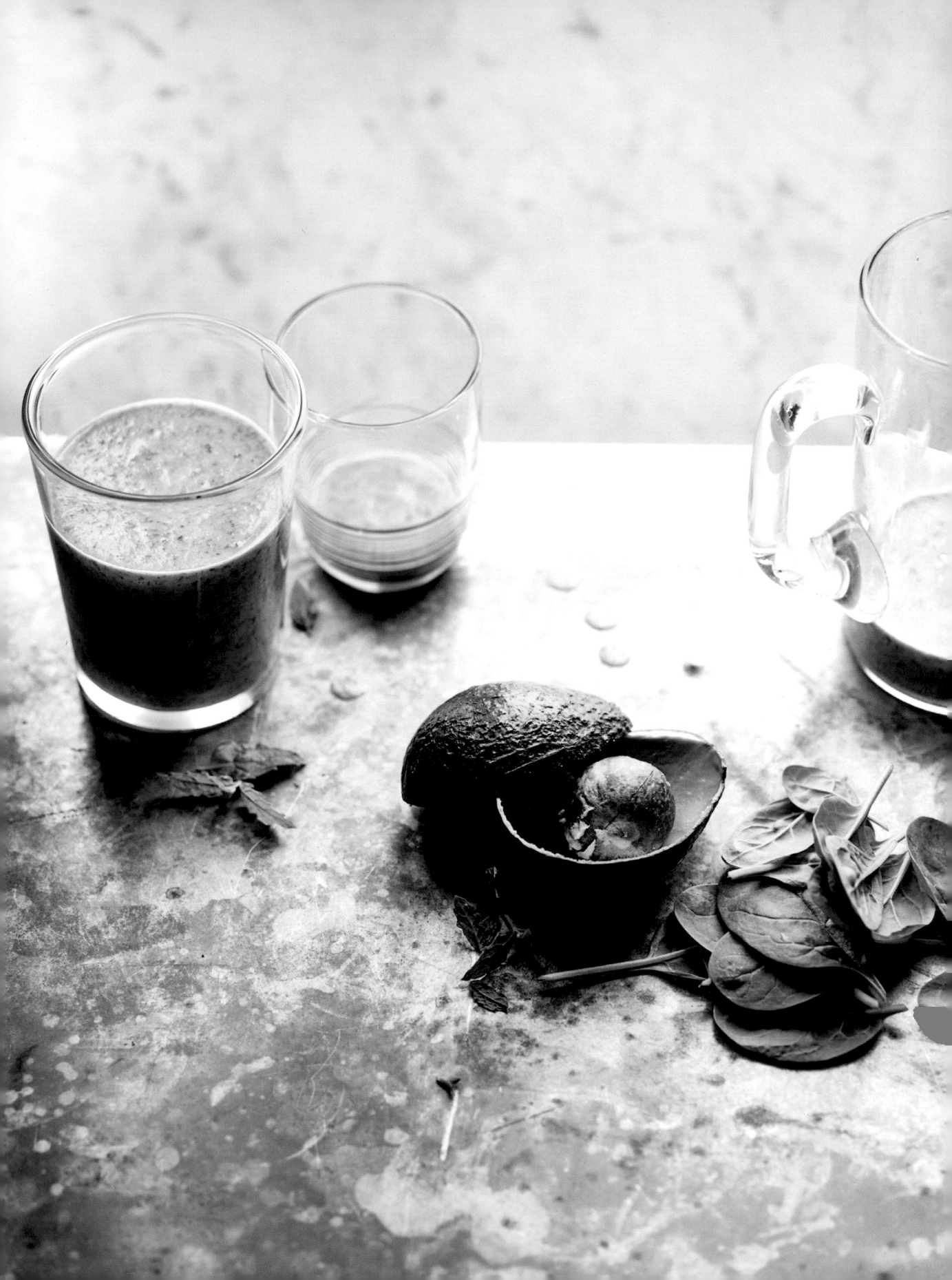

Make ahead

Crispy Bacon and Parmesan Frittata

When it comes to starting your day with healthy fats and protein, eggs are always a winner in my eyes. This is quick, easy and tastes just as good cold as it does hot.

Ingredients

3 rashers of lean smoked
  back bacon (all visible fat
  removed)
½ tbsp coconut oil
3 spring onions
salt and pepper
3 medium eggs, beaten
1 ripe plum tomato, de-seeded
  and roughly chopped
½ avocado, de-stoned and cut
  into 1.5cm pieces
1 tbsp finely grated
  parmesan cheese
rocket salad, to serve

Method

Preheat the grill to medium-high.

Place the bacon on a grill rack and cook under the grill for 2 minutes on each side until crisp. Remove from the grill and roughly chop, then place on kitchen roll to drain.

Melt the oil in an 18–20cm non-stick frying pan and add the spring onions. Stir and cook over a medium heat for 2–3 minutes. Set aside with the bacon.

Season the eggs and add to the pan. Scatter over the spring onions, tomato and the bacon.

Cook over a low to medium heat for 6–8 minutes, or until the underside is almost set.

Throw on the avocado and parmesan and place under the grill for 3–4 minutes, or until just set on the top.

Remove from the grill and allow to stand for a few minutes. Cut into wedges and serve with a rocket salad.

Reduced-carb

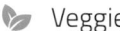 Veggie

🕐 Make ahead

Ingredients

100g baby spinach leaves
salt and pepper
30g sun-blushed tomatoes,
  drained and roughly
  chopped
40g soft goat's cheese,
  crumbled
2 medium eggs, plus
  1 medium egg white
½ tbsp coconut oil

Spinach and Goat's Cheese Omelette

Nothing beats an omelette for speed in the mornings, so ditch the sugary cereals and give this one a go. If you're not a fan of goat's cheese you could use feta or cheddar instead.

Method

Place the spinach in a pan with 2 tablespoons of water. Cover and cook for a few minutes until wilted and reduced in volume.

Remove from the heat and drain thoroughly. Chop roughly, then place it in a bowl. Season, then stir in the chopped sun-blushed tomatoes and the crumbled goat's cheese. Set aside.

In a wide bowl, whisk the whole eggs until well beaten. In a separate bowl, whisk the egg white until firm, then fold it gently but thoroughly into the beaten eggs.

Melt the oil in a 20cm non-stick frying pan and add the egg mixture. As it begins to cook, use a fork to drag the mixture into the centre, making ripples. When it is half-cooked but still runny on top, dot the spinach, tomato and cheese mixture over the surface.

Allow to cook over a medium heat for a further minute, then fold the omelette in half and cook for a bit longer, until everything is steaming and hot. You want it to remain a little runny in the centre. Slide the omelette onto a plate, and tuck in.

Reduced-carb

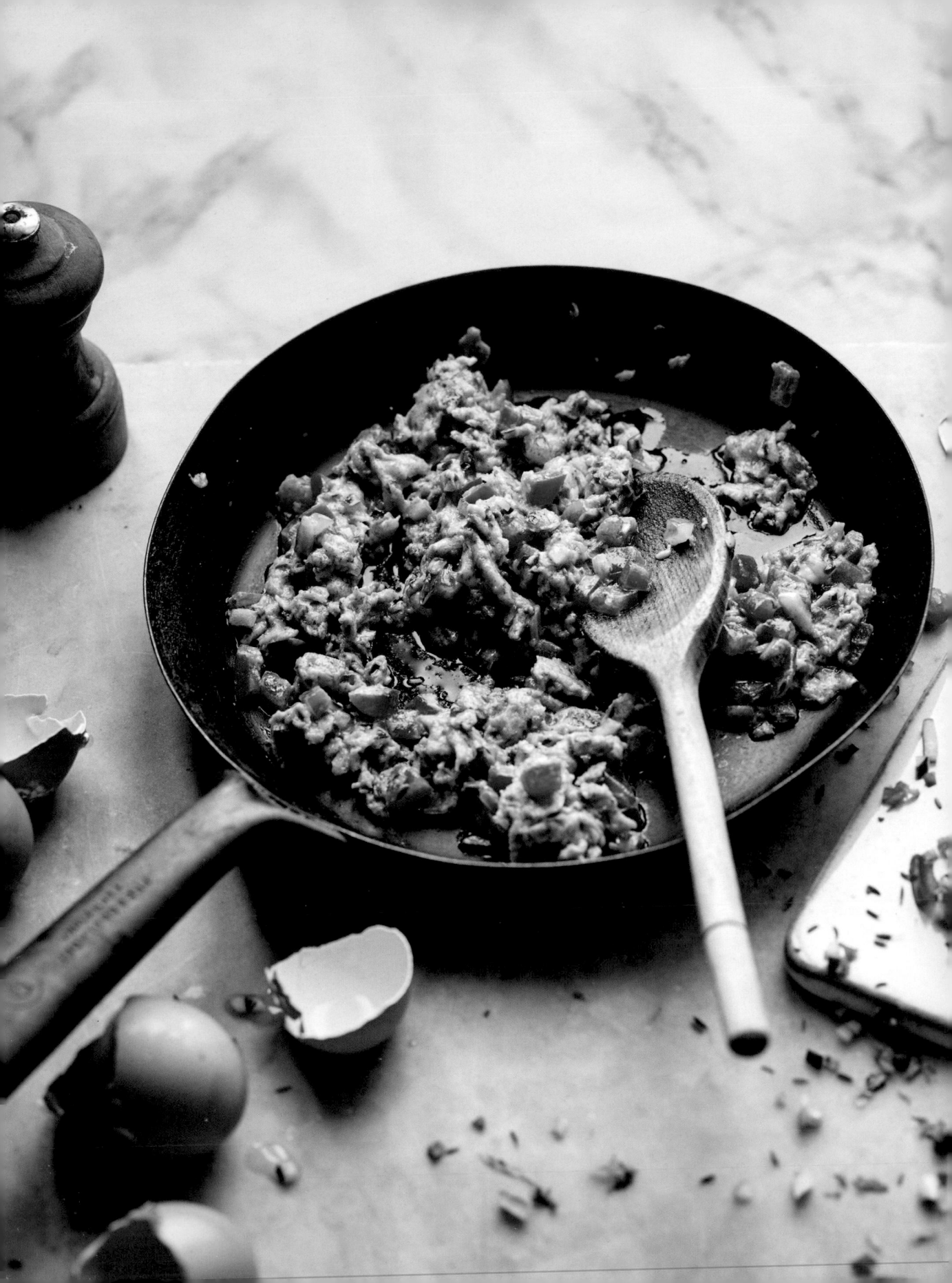

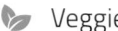 Veggie

Spicy Scrambled Eggs

Introducing the world's fastest breakfast with a spicy twist. Feel free to throw in any extra veg you have in the fridge, like spinach, kale or mixed peppers.

Ingredients

3 medium eggs
1 ripe plum tomato, de-seeded and finely chopped
2 tbsp coriander, finely chopped
1 small green chilli, de-seeded and finely chopped
salt and pepper
½ tbsp coconut oil
½ red onion, finely diced
1 tsp cumin seeds
1 tsp ground turmeric

Method

Place the eggs in a bowl and lightly beat them. Stir in the tomato, coriander and green chilli until well combined. Season well.

Melt the oil in a medium non-stick frying pan over a gentle heat. Add the onion and cumin and stir-fry for 2–3 minutes until softened.

Stir in the turmeric, then pour in the egg mixture and scramble over a gentle heat for 1–2 minutes, or until cooked to your liking.

Remove from the heat and serve.

Reduced-carb

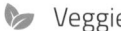 Veggie

Ingredients

30g quinoa
100g feta cheese, crumbled
2 spring onions, very finely chopped
1 clove garlic, crushed
1 tsp sweet smoked paprika
2 large eggs
salt and pepper
1 tbsp coconut oil
1 long red chilli, de-seeded and finely chopped
1 tbsp flat-leaf parsley, finely chopped

Quinoa and Feta Fritter with Poached Egg

This is a simple but very tasty breakfast idea. The quinoa and feta cheese work so well together. Enjoy!

Method

Cook the quinoa according to packet instructions.

Place the cooked quinoa, feta, spring onions, garlic and sweet smoked paprika into a food processor. Lightly beat one of the eggs and add to the mixture. Blend until well combined and season well.

Melt the oil in a 12cm non-stick frying pan and preheat the grill to medium to hot. Add the quinoa mixture and press down with the back of a spoon to make a smooth cake. Fry for 3–4 minutes, then place under the grill and cook for 3–4 minutes, or until set and golden.

Meanwhile, poach the remaining egg: bring a pan of water to a gentle boil and crack in the egg. Poach at a gentle simmer for 3–4 minutes, or until cooked to your liking.

Top the quinoa fritter with the poached egg and top with the red chilli and parsley.

Reduced-carb

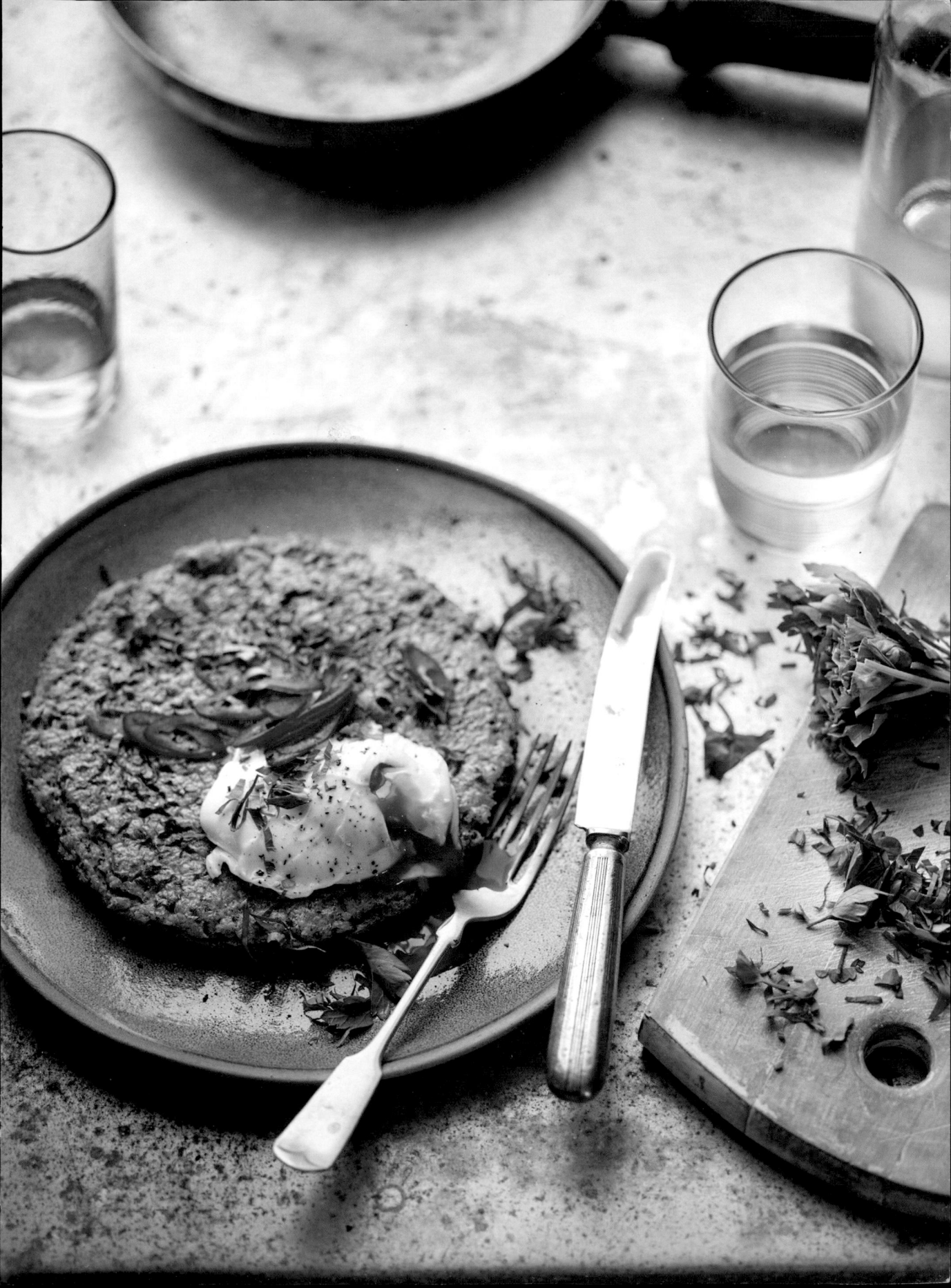

Veggie

Turkish-style Eggs with Roasted Peppers and Yoghurt

Ooooh talk about flavours! This is easily my favourite reduced-carb breakfast in the book. A true Lean in 15 recipe, this is not to be missed.

Ingredients

100g Greek-style yoghurt
1 clove garlic, crushed
1 tsp finely grated lemon zest
1 tsp lemon juice
salt and pepper
100g baby spinach leaves
1 tbsp olive oil
2 jarred red peppers,
  roughly chopped
2 medium eggs
1 tbsp unsalted butter
½ tsp dried aleppo or dried
  red chilli flakes
½ tsp sweet smoked paprika
1 tbsp mint leaves (optional)

Method

Mix the yoghurt, garlic, lemon zest and juice in a small bowl, season and set aside.

Wilt the spinach in a saucepan of boiling water for 1 minute. Drain the spinach, squeeze out the excess water and season.

Warm the oil in a 14cm non-stick frying pan over a medium heat. Add the spinach to the pan with the chopped peppers, spreading them evenly over the base.

Make two wells in the mixture and crack an egg into each. Cook for 5–6 minutes, so that the yolks are still soft, covering the pan with a lid for the last 2 minutes to set the whites.

In a small pan, heat the butter until foaming. Swirl in the aleppo or chilli flakes, paprika and a pinch of salt and cook for a couple of seconds, then take off the heat.

Drizzle the yoghurt mixture over the eggs, then top with the chilli butter and serve, scattered with the mint leaves, if using.

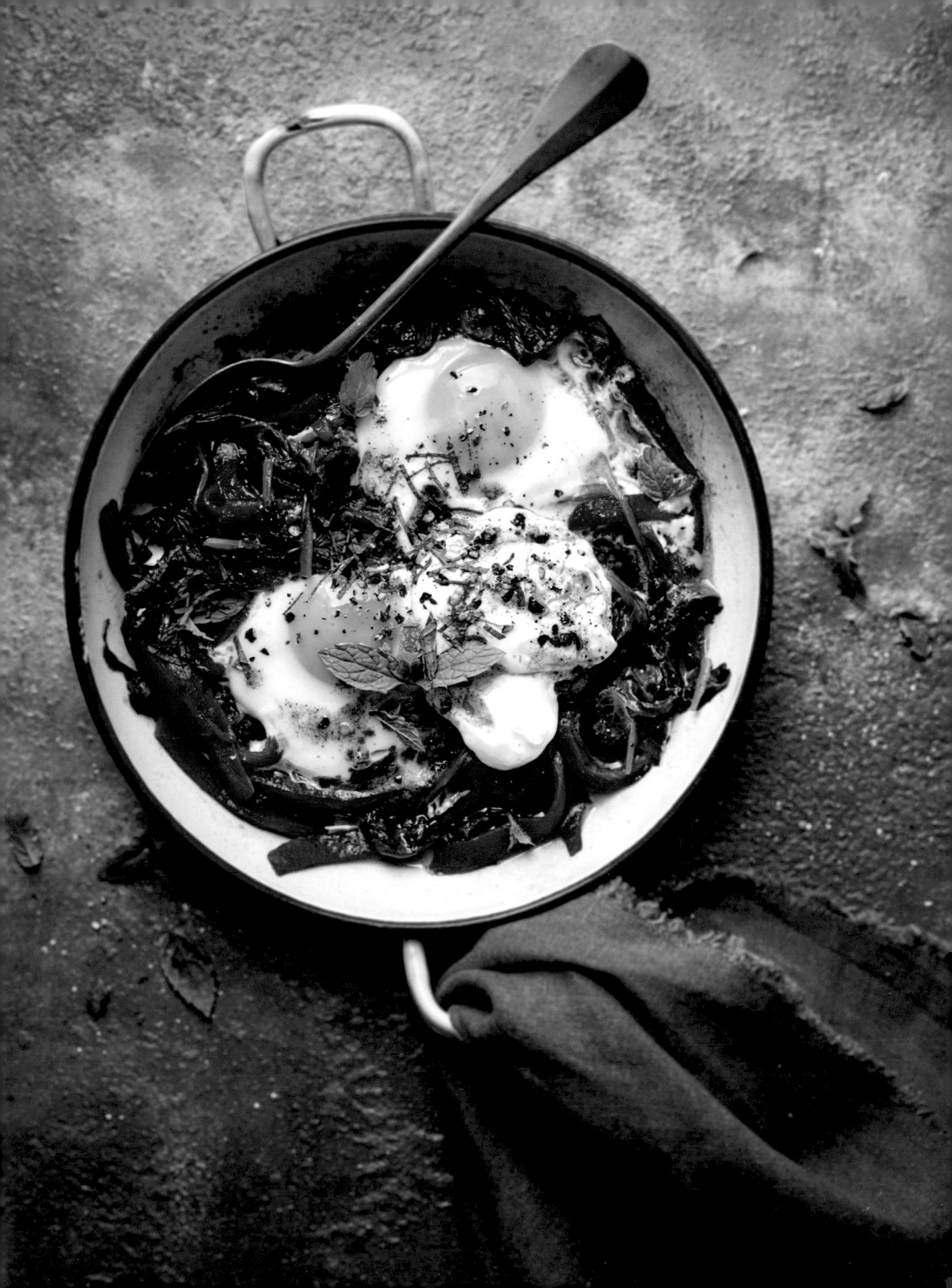

Thai Chicken Lettuce Wraps

I'm absolutely obsessed with this recipe. If you love Thai flavours, be sure to try this. You'll be making it over and over again.

Ingredients

1 x 200g skinless chicken breast or thigh fillet, roughly chopped
2 tbsp coriander (stalks and leaves), finely chopped
1 tsp finely chopped mint
1 tsp lemongrass paste
2 spring onions, finely chopped
zest and juice of 1 lime
salt and pepper
1 tomato, diced
¼ cucumber, diced
2 tbsp coarsely grated carrot
3 romaine lettuce leaves
1–2 tbsp sweet chilli sauce
2 tbsp roasted peanuts, roughly chopped

Method

Preheat the grill to high.

Place the chicken in a food processor with the coriander, mint, lemongrass paste, spring onions and lime zest. Season with salt and pepper and pulse until well combined.

Divide the mixture into nine balls. Place the balls on a grill rack over a baking tray and grill for 4–5 minutes on each side, or until browned and cooked through.

While the balls are cooking, mix together the cucumber, tomato and carrot in a bowl and stir in the lime juice. Season and toss to mix well.

To serve, place the lettuce leaves on a serving plate and top with the cucumber mixture. Divide the chicken balls between them, and top with the sweet chilli sauce and chopped peanuts.

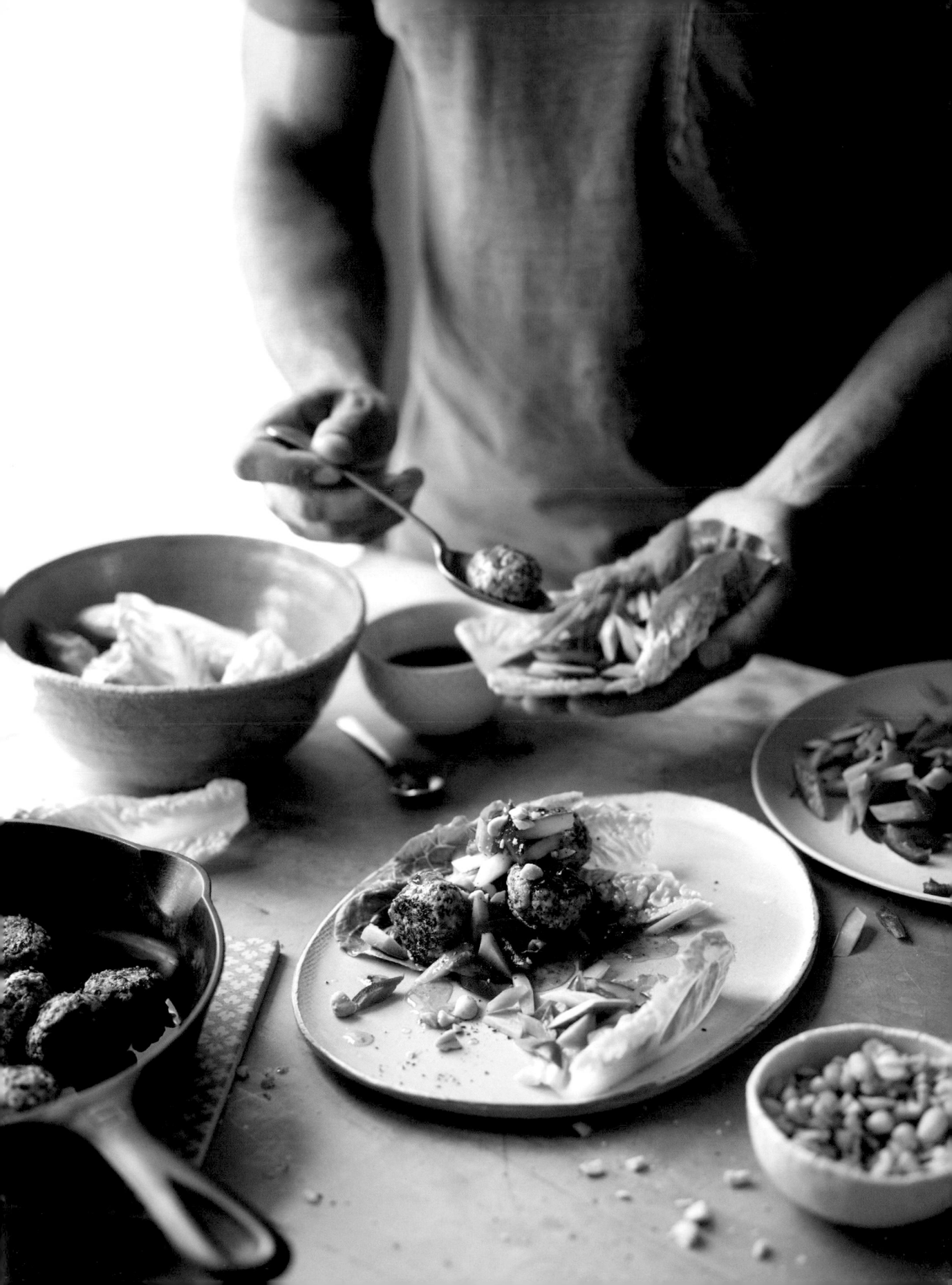

Veggie
 Make ahead

Ingredients

1 tbsp coconut oil

1 x 250g pack pre-cooked
puy lentils

¼ x 400g tin of chickpeas,
drained

75ml very hot vegetable stock

2 cooked beetroots, finely
chopped

¼ fennel bulb, cored and very
thinly sliced

2 tbsp mint, very finely
chopped

2 tbsp coriander, very finely
chopped

1 tbsp apple cider vinegar

juice of ½ orange

50g midget trees (tenderstem
broccoli), thinly sliced

salt and pepper

½ ripe avocado, de-stoned

30g feta cheese, crumbled

1 tbsp toasted pumpkin seeds
(optional)

1 tbsp pomegranate seeds
(optional)

Joe's Veggie Super Bowl

Here's a vegetarian meal that is packed full of goodness
and flavour. It makes a great lunch on the go, so box it up
and carry it to work for the win.

Method

Melt the coconut oil in a wide non-stick saucepan and
add the lentils, chickpeas and stock.

Stir and cook for 3–4 minutes over a high heat, or until
the stock is absorbed.

Chuck in the the beetroots and fennel and remove the
pan from the heat. Stir in the chopped herbs, vinegar
and orange juice.

In a small saucepan of lightly salted boiling water, blanch
the midget trees for 2 minutes, then drain and add into
the quinoa mixture. Season and toss to mix well.

Place a non-stick griddle pan on a high heat and when hot
add the avocado, cut side-down. Griddle for 3 minutes.

Place the quinoa mixture in a wide bowl, top with the
griddled avocado and scatter with feta and the pumpkin
and pomegranate seeds, if using. Season and serve.

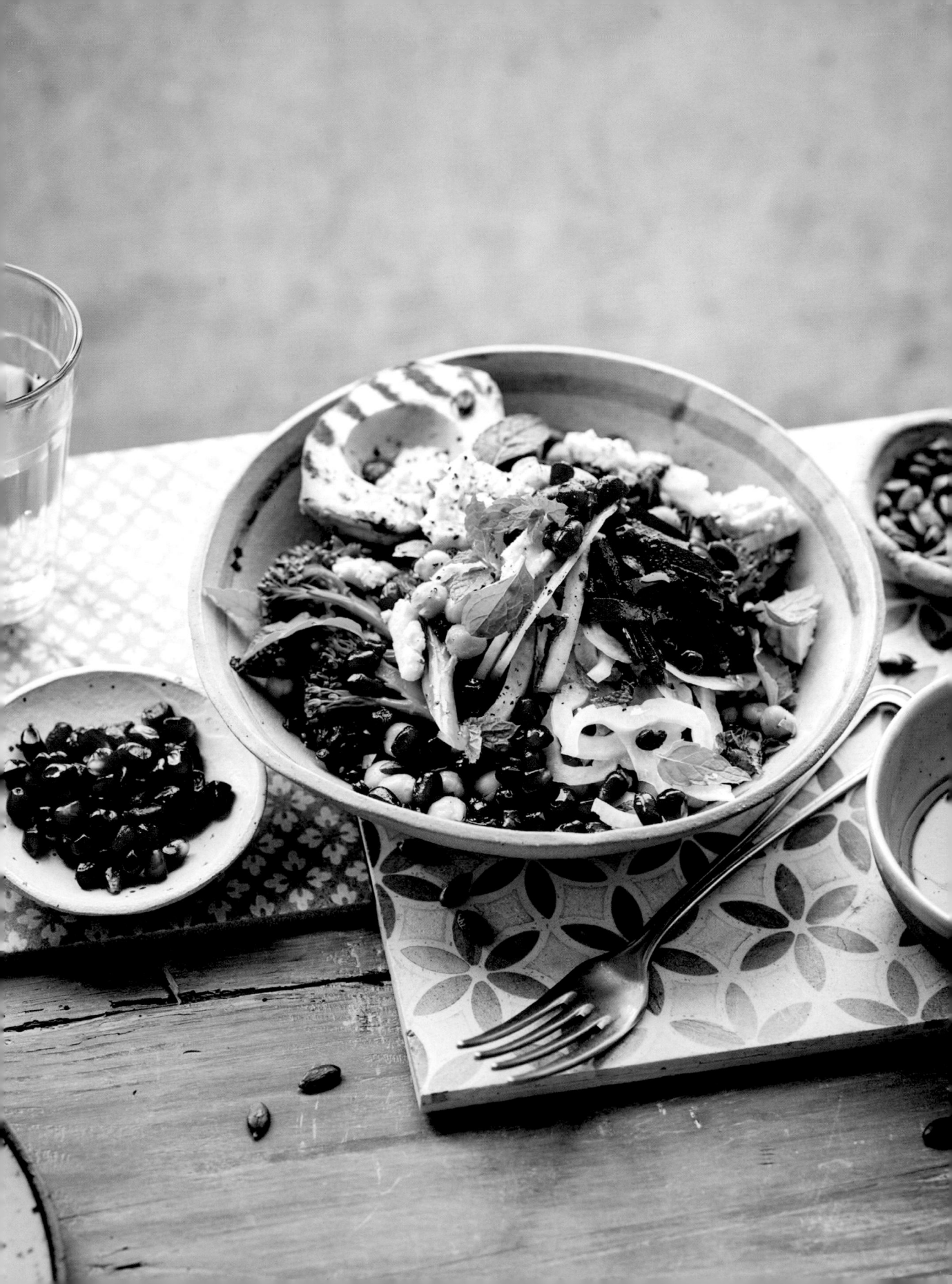

Beefy Butternut Squash with Mascarpone

I know I'm lazy here, using ready-made butternut squash noodles, but they're hassle-free and make a great alternative to spaghetti or egg noodles. I think you'll be surprised at how good this one tastes and how much it fills you up.

Ingredients

1 tbsp coconut oil
180g extra-lean beef
  steak mince
2 cloves garlic, crushed
½ tsp dried red chilli flakes
½ x 400g tin of
  chopped tomatoes
2 tbsp tomato puree
salt and pepper
large handful of basil,
  chopped, plus extra
  for garnish
50g mascarpone cheese
200g ready-made butternut
  squash noodles or courgetti

Method

Melt the oil in a wide non-stick frying pan over a medium heat. Add the beef mince and stir-fry for 3–4 minutes, or until sealed and browned.

Stir in the garlic, chilli flakes, tomatoes and tomato puree. Stir and cook over a medium heat for 6–8 minutes or until bubbling. Season well, remove from the heat and stir in the basil and the mascarpone. Cover and keep warm.

Cook the butternut squash noodles according to packet instructions, and pile them onto a warmed serving bowl or plate. Spoon over the beefy sauce and top with basil leaves before serving.

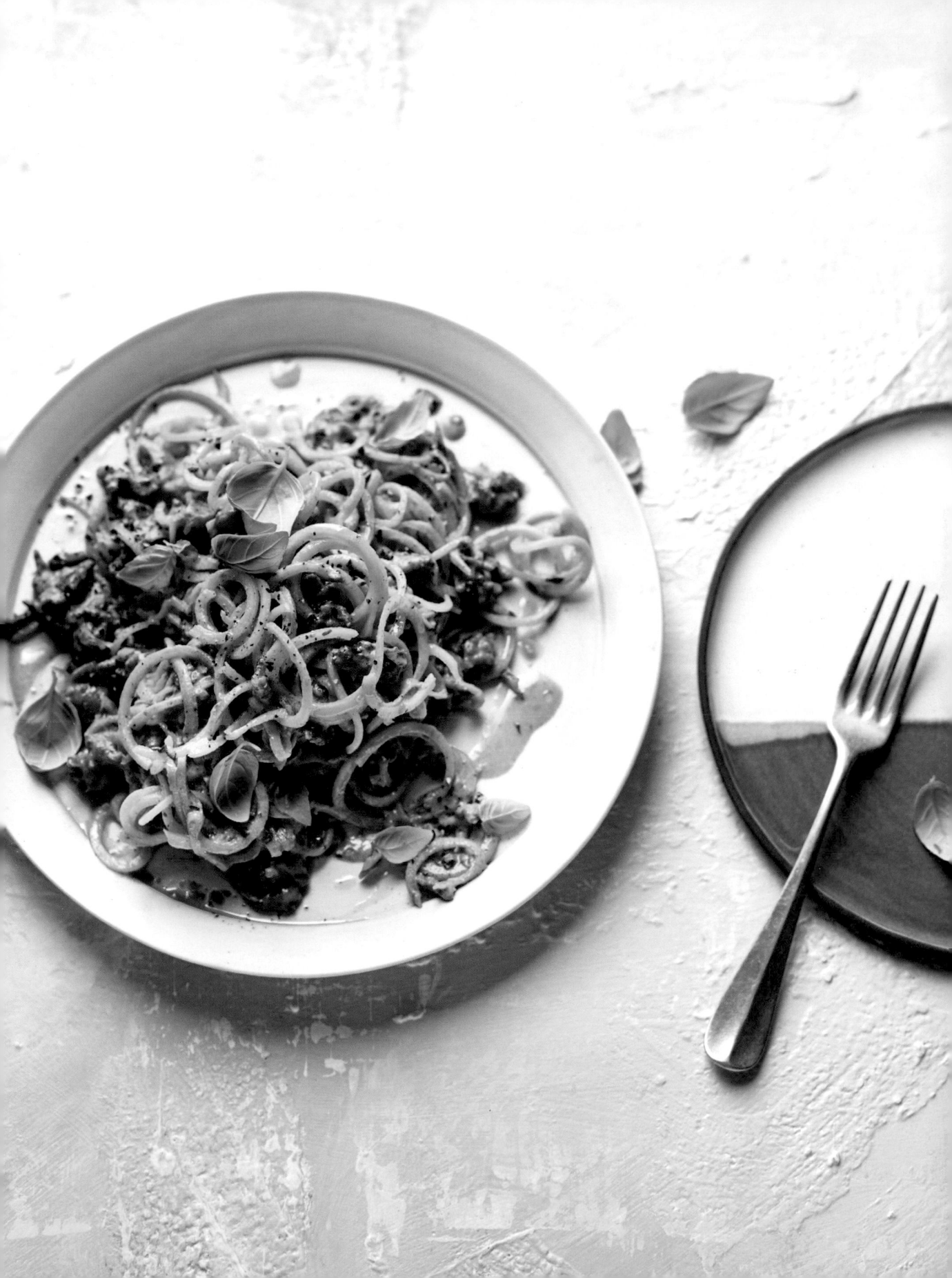

Tandoori Chicken with Cauliflower Pilau Rice

Next time you fancy ordering a take-away curry, put down the phone and grab this recipe instead. It's going to satisfy your cravings and keep you bang on track to staying lean.

Ingredients

1 x 180g skinless chicken breast fillet
2 tsp tandoori or tikka spice mix
1 clove garlic, crushed or finely grated
juice of ½ lime
salt and pepper

For the pilau 'rice'

200g cauliflower florets
1 tbsp coconut oil
1 banana shallot, finely chopped
1½ tbsp pilau spice mix
250g frozen mixed vegetables
4 tbsp coriander, chopped, plus extra sprigs to serve
lime wedges, to serve

Method

Place the chicken between two pieces of cling film, and using a rolling pin or wooden mallet, lightly beat until about 1cm thick.

Mix the spice mix with the garlic and lime juice and spread all over the chicken. Season lightly with salt and slide onto a grill rack.

While the chicken is marinating, make the pilau 'rice'. Blitz the cauliflower in a food processor until it resembles rice.

Melt the coconut oil in a wide non-stick frying pan and add the shallot, cauliflower and pilau spice mix. Stir-fry for 1–2 minutes on a high heat.

Add the frozen mixed vegetables and a splash of boiling water, and continue to stir-fry for 6–7 minutes, or until piping hot. Remove from the heat, stir in the coriander, cover and keep warm.

Preheat the grill to high.

Place the chicken under the grill and cook for 3 minutes on each side, or until cooked through. Check by slicing into it to make sure the meat is white all the way through, with no raw pink bits left. Remove from the grill and roughly slice into strips.

Plate up the pilau 'rice' and top with the chicken. Serve with wedges of lime and coriander sprigs.

Reduced-carb

Make ahead

Lamb and Coconut Curry

You don't need loads of rice and naan bread to enjoy a curry. This low-carb version will hit the spot and keep you on track to reaching your goals. The lamb mince and coconut flavours work perfectly here.

Ingredients

1 tbsp coconut oil
1 small onion, finely chopped
1 carrot, cut into 1cm dice
200g lean lamb mince
1 clove garlic, crushed
1 tsp finely grated ginger
1 red chilli, de-seeded and finely chopped
2 tbsp medium curry paste
2 tbsp coconut cream
½ x 400g tin of chopped tomatoes
200g frozen peas
large handful of coriander, chopped, plus extra sprigs for garnish

Method

Melt the oil in a large pan. Add the onion, carrot and lamb mince and cook for 5 minutes until softened.

Stir in the garlic, ginger, chilli, curry paste, coconut cream and chopped tomatoes. Stir and cook over a high heat for 8–10 minutes, adding the peas for the last 2–3 minutes.

Remove from the heat and stir in the coriander. Transfer to a bowl and top with extra coriander sprigs.

Reduced-carb

Make ahead

Beetroot, Feta and Chicken Salad

If you're looking for a quick recipe to take to work for lunch then this is ideal. It contains protein and healthy fats to fuel your body and provides you with plenty of energy.

Ingredients

1 x 200g skinless chicken
  breast or thigh fillet
½ tbsp coconut oil
20g rocket leaves
200g cooked beetroot
100g feta cheese, crumbled
1 long red chilli, de-seeded and
  very finely chopped
small handful of mint,
  chopped
small handful of parsley,
  chopped (optional)
2 spring onions, finely sliced
1 tbsp apple cider vinegar
juice of ½ orange
1 tbsp Dijon mustard
salt and pepper

Method

Place the chicken between two pieces of cling film, and using a rolling pin or wooden mallet, lightly beat until slightly thinned to an even thickness.

Melt the coconut oil on a hot griddle pan and cook the chicken for 6–8 minutes on each side, until cooked through. Check by slicing into it to make sure the meat is white all the way through, with no raw pink bits left.

Scatter the rocket leaves on a serving plate. Cut the beetroot into wedges and scatter them over the rocket.

Roughly tear the chicken into bite-sized pieces and sprinkle over the beetroot. Scatter over the feta, chilli, mint, parsley (if using) and spring onions.

Mix together the vinegar, orange juice and mustard in a small jug. Season well and drizzle over the salad. Toss to mix well and tuck in.

Tip This recipe uses cooked beetroot but you could cook your own beetroot up to 3 days in advance – simply wrap it in foil and roast in a hot oven for 40–60 minutes (depending on the size) until tender when pierced with a skewer. When cool, peel and use as above.

Reduced-carb

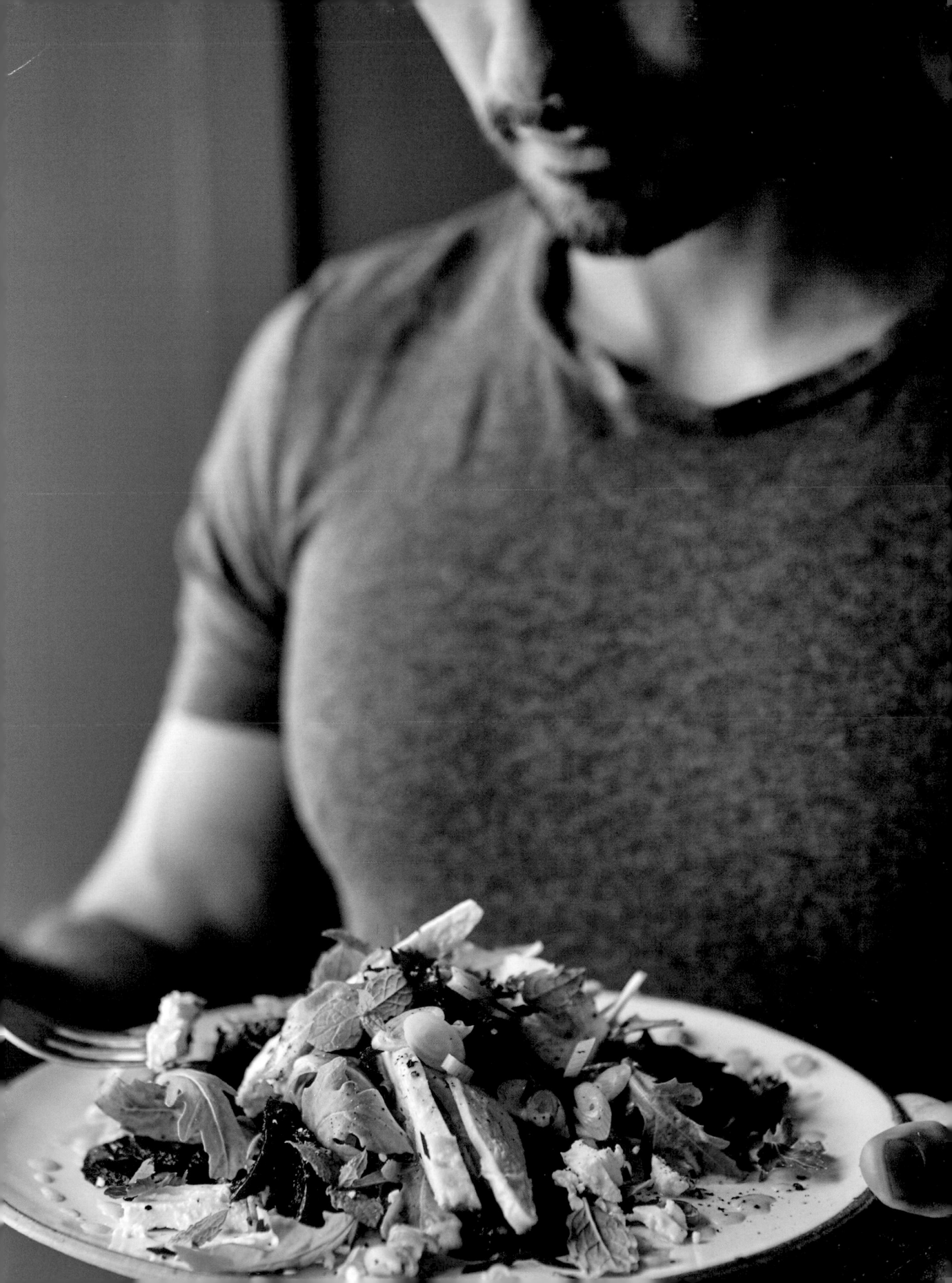

Make ahead

Asian Beef Stir-fry with Oyster Sauce

This is a one-wok wonder that is packed full of flavour and goodness. It makes a great lunch for work so you could double up the recipe.

Ingredients

1 tbsp coconut oil
1 lean sirloin or fillet steak, thinly sliced
1 tbsp ginger, finely grated
1 tbsp garlic, finely grated
2 spring onions, diagonally sliced into 3cm lengths
150g shiitake mushrooms, thinly sliced
100g choi sum or pak choi, roughly sliced
50g mangetout, trimmed
2 tbsp oyster sauce
1 tbsp dark soy sauce
2 tbsp toasted cashews, roughly chopped

Method

Melt half of the oil in a large non-stick wok or wide non-stick frying pan over a high heat. Add the slices of steak and stir-fry for 1–2 minutes until sealed and lightly browned. Transfer to a plate.

Place the wok over a medium heat and add the remaining oil. Stir in the ginger, garlic and spring onions, and stir-fry for 1 minute.

Increase the heat to high and add the mushrooms, choi sum or pak choi and mangetout. Stir and toss together for 3–4 minutes. Return the steak to the pan with the oyster sauce and soy sauce. Toss and stir-fry for 2–3 minutes.

Transfer to a bowl and serve topped with the cashews.

Reduced-carb

Citrus Salmon with Minty Bean Salad

The lemon and mint in this recipe taste so fresh with the salmon. I'm sure you'll enjoy this time and time again.

Ingredients

1 tbsp coconut oil
1 x 180g salmon fillet, skin-on
salt and pepper
juice of ½ lemon, plus extra
  wedges for garnish
250g green beans, trimmed
1 large clove garlic,
  thinly sliced
1 ripe plum tomato,
  finely diced
1 tbsp balsamic vinegar
2 tbsp mint, finely chopped

Method

Melt half of the oil in a non-stick frying pan. Add the salmon skin-side down, season with salt and pepper and squeeze over a little lemon juice.

Fry for 3–4 minutes, then turn the salmon over and fry for a further 1–2 minutes, or until cooked through. Squeeze over a little more lemon juice and season to taste. Remove from the pan and set aside.

Meanwhile, cook the beans in boiling salted water for 5–6 minutes, until just tender, then drain.

Melt the remaining oil in a small frying pan, add the garlic and stir-fry quickly until crisp and lightly golden. Remove from the heat and add the tomato.

Whisk together the balsamic and mint, and season well. Pour over the beans and mix well.

Tip into a serving bowl and scatter over the tomato and garlic mixture. Place the salmon on top and serve with extra lemon wedges.

Reduced-carb

Prawn and Avocado Salad with Miso Soy Dressing

The dressing for this salad tastes incredible and can be made up to 3 days in advance. Just store it in the fridge and give it a good shake before using.

Ingredients

¼ cucumber
½ ripe avocado, de-stoned
25g baby spinach leaves
5 red radishes, thinly sliced
50g red and yellow cherry tomatoes, halved
1 carrot, grated
50g sugarsnap peas, finely sliced lengthways
150g cooked peeled tiger prawns

For the miso soy dressing

50ml mirin
1 tsp miso paste
juice of ½ orange
¼ tsp finely grated ginger
¼ tsp toasted sesame oil
juice of 1 lime
1 tbsp light soy sauce
¼ tsp English mustard

Method

Place all of the dressing ingredients in a clean, screw-top jam jar.

Peel the cucumber into thin ribbons using a vegetable peeler. Thinly slice the avocado. Place the spinach and chopped vegetables in a wide bowl and top with the prawns.

Shake the dressing in the jam jar until well mixed and pour over the salad. Toss the whole lot together and enjoy.

Reduced-carb

5-spice Hoisin Chicken Skewers

These skewers with Asian mushrooms and greens are perfect any day of the week. Pull them out at your next barbecue to impress your friends.

Ingredients

1 x 200g skinless chicken
  breast fillet, cut into
  2.5cm pieces
2 tbsp hoisin sauce
2 tbsp light soy sauce
½ tbsp sweet chilli sauce
½ tsp 5-spice mix
½ tbsp coconut oil
10g fresh ginger, cut into thin
  matchsticks or finely grated
4 spring onions, cut into
  4cm diagonal lengths
½ red pepper, de-seeded and
  thinly sliced
250g assorted Asian
  mushrooms (oyster, enoki or
  shiitake), sliced if large
250g baby pak choi, halved
  or quartered

Method

Place the chicken in a stainless-steel, ceramic or glass bowl. Mix together the hoisin, soy sauce, sweet chilli sauce and 5-spice and drizzle half the mixture over the chicken, tossing to coat well.

Preheat the grill to medium-high.

Thread the chicken pieces onto two metal or pre-soaked bamboo skewers. Place the skewers on a grill rack under the grill and cook for 6–8 minutes, turning halfway through, until cooked through and lightly browned.

Meanwhile, melt the oil in a wide non-stick frying pan over a medium to high heat. Add the ginger, spring onions, red pepper and mushrooms and stir-fry for 3–4 minutes. Add the baby pak choi and stir-fry for 3 minutes, or until just tender.

Add the sauce mixture and cook until everything is coated and heated through. Serve in a wide bowl, topped with the chicken skewers.

Reduced-carb

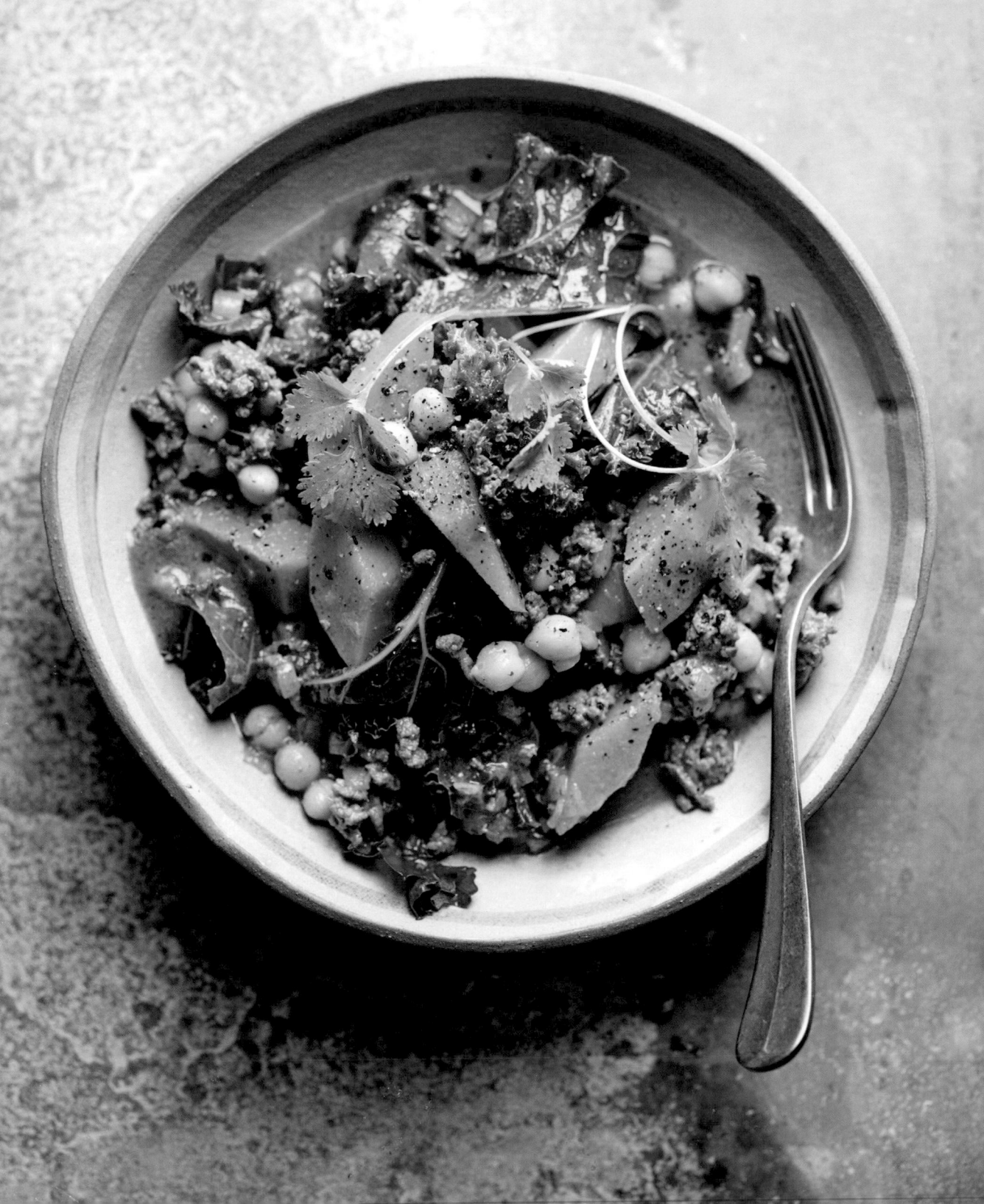

Beef, Butternut and Coconut Stew

I love the flavours in this recipe. It's so satisfying and will really fill you up. Be sure to remove the skin from the butternut squash and chop it into tiny cubes so it cooks faster.

Ingredients

½ tbsp coconut oil
180g extra-lean beef
  steak mince
1 onion, finely diced
1½ tbsp Thai red curry paste
250g butternut squash or
  sweet potato, peeled and cut
  into 1cm cubes
½ x 400g tin of chickpeas,
  rinsed and drained
100g coconut cream
400ml fresh chicken or
  vegetable stock
50g shredded kale
large handful of chopped
  coriander, chopped,
  plus extra for garnish
juice of 1 lime

Method

Melt the oil in a wide non-stick frying pan over a high heat. Add the beef mince and onion and stir-fry for 3–4 minutes.

Stir in the curry paste, butternut squash or sweet potato and chickpeas and stir-fry for 1–2 minutes.

Add the coconut cream and stock and bring to a fast boil. Cover and cook for 6–8 minutes over a high heat and then add the kale and coriander.

Continue to cook for 2–3 minutes, or until the butternut squash or sweet potato is tender, then remove from the heat.

Ladle into a warmed serving bowl, stir in the lime juice and top with sprigs of coriander.

Reduced-carb

🕑 Make ahead

Grilled Harissa Chicken and Chickpea Salad

If you've not tasted harissa paste before, this is your chance. It's one of my favourite flavours. You can find it in most supermarkets now – use it with fish, chicken or beef.

Ingredients

200g mini chicken fillets (or 1 x 200g chicken breast fillet, cut into strips)
1 tbsp harissa paste
finely grated zest and juice of 1 lemon
1 clove garlic, crushed
salt and pepper
50g midget trees (tenderstem broccoli), thinly sliced
½ tbsp coconut oil
2 spring onions, finely sliced
3 jarred red peppers, roughly chopped
½ x 400g tin of chickpeas, rinsed and drained
2 small handfuls of baby spinach leaves
small handful each of coriander, flat-leaf parsley and mint leaves, chopped
1 tbsp pomegranate seeds (optional)
1 tbsp toasted pine nuts (optional)

Method

Place the chicken fillets in a stainless-steel, ceramic or glass bowl. Mix together the harissa paste, lemon zest and garlic and use it to coat the chicken. Season with salt.

Meanwhile, blanch the broccoli in a small saucepan of boiling hot water for 2–3 minutes, or until just tender. Drain and transfer to a mixing bowl. Preheat the grill to medium-high.

Slide the chicken onto a grill rack and place under the grill. Cook for 5–6 minutes, turning halfway through, until cooked through. Check by slicing into one of the pieces to make sure the meat is white all the way through, with no raw pink bits left.

Meanwhile, melt the oil in a non-stick frying pan and add the spring onions, peppers, chickpeas and spinach. Season, toss to mix well, and stir and cook for 3–4 minutes until the spinach is wilted.

Remove the pan from the heat and stir in the lemon juice and chopped herbs. Toss to mix well and pile onto a serving plate, topped with the grilled chicken. Scatter over the pomegranate seeds and pine nuts, if using, and serve warm, or at room temperature.

Reduced-carb

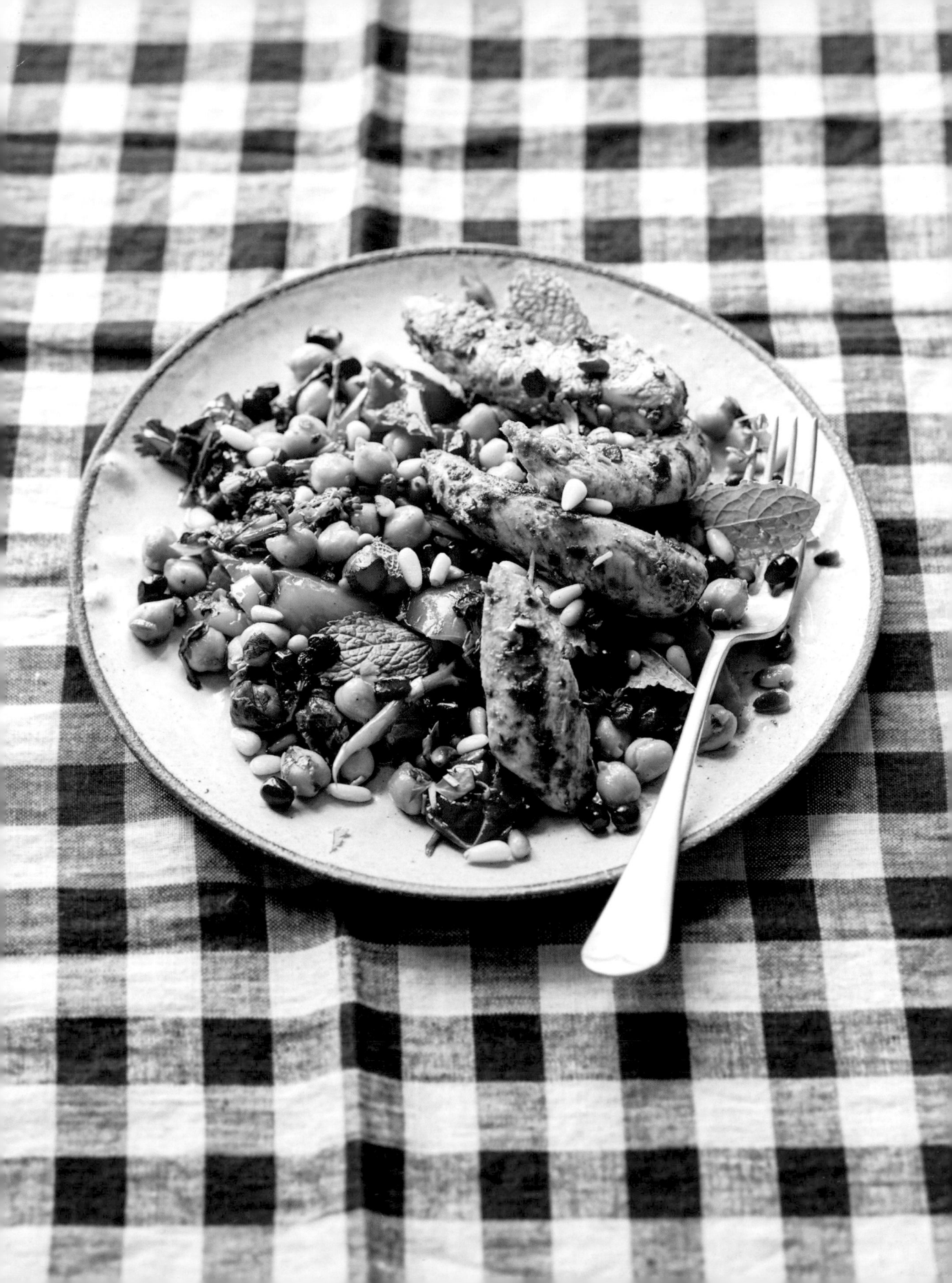

Griddled Tuna Steak with Midget Trees

Just in case you're wondering, 'midget trees' is my name for broccoli. This dish comes with a really tasty dressing, too.

Ingredients

- 100g midget trees (tenderstem broccoli), cut into short lengths
- 100g green beans, halved
- 2 tbsp parsley, finely chopped
- 2 tbsp finely chopped cornichons or gherkins
- 2 tsp capers, rinsed and drained
- 1 red chilli, finely chopped – remove the seeds if you don't like it hot
- 1 clove garlic, finely chopped
- 1 ripe, plum tomato, finely chopped
- zest of ½ lemon
- 1 tbsp apple cider vinegar
- 1 tsp dijon mustard
- 50g pre-cooked puy lentils
- salt and pepper
- 1 x 200g tuna steak
- 1 tbsp toasted sesame seeds (optional)

Method

Boil the broccoli and green beans in a small saucepan of boiling water for 2–3 minutes, or until just tender. Drain and place in a mixing bowl.

Chuck in the parsley, cornichons or gherkins, capers, red chilli, garlic, tomato, lemon zest, vinegar, mustard and lentils. Season well with salt and black pepper and toss to mix well.

Meanwhile, heat a non-stick, ridged griddle pan until smoking and add the tuna. Cook for 1–2 minutes on each side, or until cooked to your liking. The less you cook the tuna, the more moist it will be!

Heap the broccoli mixture onto a serving plate and top with the tuna. Season, scatter over the sesame seeds, if using, and serve.

Tip For a bigger citrussy flavour, add 1 tablespoon of grated orange zest to the lentil mixture as well.

Maple-glazed Lamb Chops with Creamy Kale

I'm feeling quite sad that there's no image to entice you with this recipe, but take my word for it when I say this is probably the tastiest thing I've ever made.

Ingredients

3 lean lamb chops or cutlets
salt and pepper
1 tbsp balsamic vinegar
1 tbsp maple syrup
¼ tsp ground cinnamon
150g shredded kale
1 tbsp coconut oil
½ red onion, finely diced
2 cloves garlic, crushed
2 tsp wholegrain mustard
70ml chicken stock
30ml double cream

Method

Preheat the grill to medium. Season the chops with salt and pepper on both sides. Cook under the grill for 4–5 minutes on each side, or until cooked to your liking.

To make the glaze, mix the balsamic, syrup and cinnamon together. Remove the chops from the grill and brush with the glaze on both sides. Return and cook for a further 1–2 minutes on each side.

Meanwhile, make the creamed kale by placing the kale in a saucepan of boiling water. Boil for 2–3 minutes, then drain completely, squeezing out any liquid.

Melt the oil in a wide non-stick frying pan and add the red onion and garlic. Stir-fry over a medium heat for 2–3 minutes and then add the kale, mustard, stock and cream. Bring to the boil and simmer for 2–3 minutes.

Season well and remove from the heat. Spoon the creamed kale onto a serving plate and top with the glazed lamb chops.

Reduced-carb

Sweet 'n' Sticky Chicken with Bean and Lentil Salad

Mmm sticky chicken … Yes please! This recipe has so many awesome flavours going on. It will work well as a lunch on the go, too.

Ingredients

1 x 180g skinless chicken breast fillet
½ tbsp balsamic vinegar
½ tbsp dark soy sauce
½ tbsp sweet chilli sauce
1 tsp finely grated ginger
3 tbsp mint, finely chopped
100g podded broad beans (thawed if frozen)
large fistful of lamb's lettuce
75g pre-cooked puy lentils
6 cherry tomatoes, halved
¼ cucumber, diced
½ tbsp wholegrain mustard
1 tbsp apple cider vinegar
1 tbsp fresh orange juice
salt and pepper

Method

Place the chicken between two pieces of cling film and using a rolling pin or mallet, lightly beat the thickest part of the breast until the whole thing is about 1.5cm thick.

Cut the chicken into three pieces and place in a bowl with the balsamic, soy sauce, sweet chilli sauce, ginger and 1 teaspoon of the mint. Toss to mix well.

Meanwhile, bring a small pan of water to the boil. Drop in the broad beans and cook them for 2 minutes. Drain and slip the beans from their skins, then place in a wide mixing bowl.

Heat a non-stick, ridged griddle pan until hot and add the chicken. Cook for 2–3 minutes on each side, or until lightly charred, sticky and cooked through. Check by slicing into it to make sure the meat is white all the way through, with no raw pink bits left, then cut it up into thin slices.

Toss the broad beans with the lamb's lettuce, lentils, tomatoes, cucumber and the remaining mint together with the mustard, apple cider vinegar and orange juice. Season well and serve with the warm, sticky chicken.

Reduced-carb

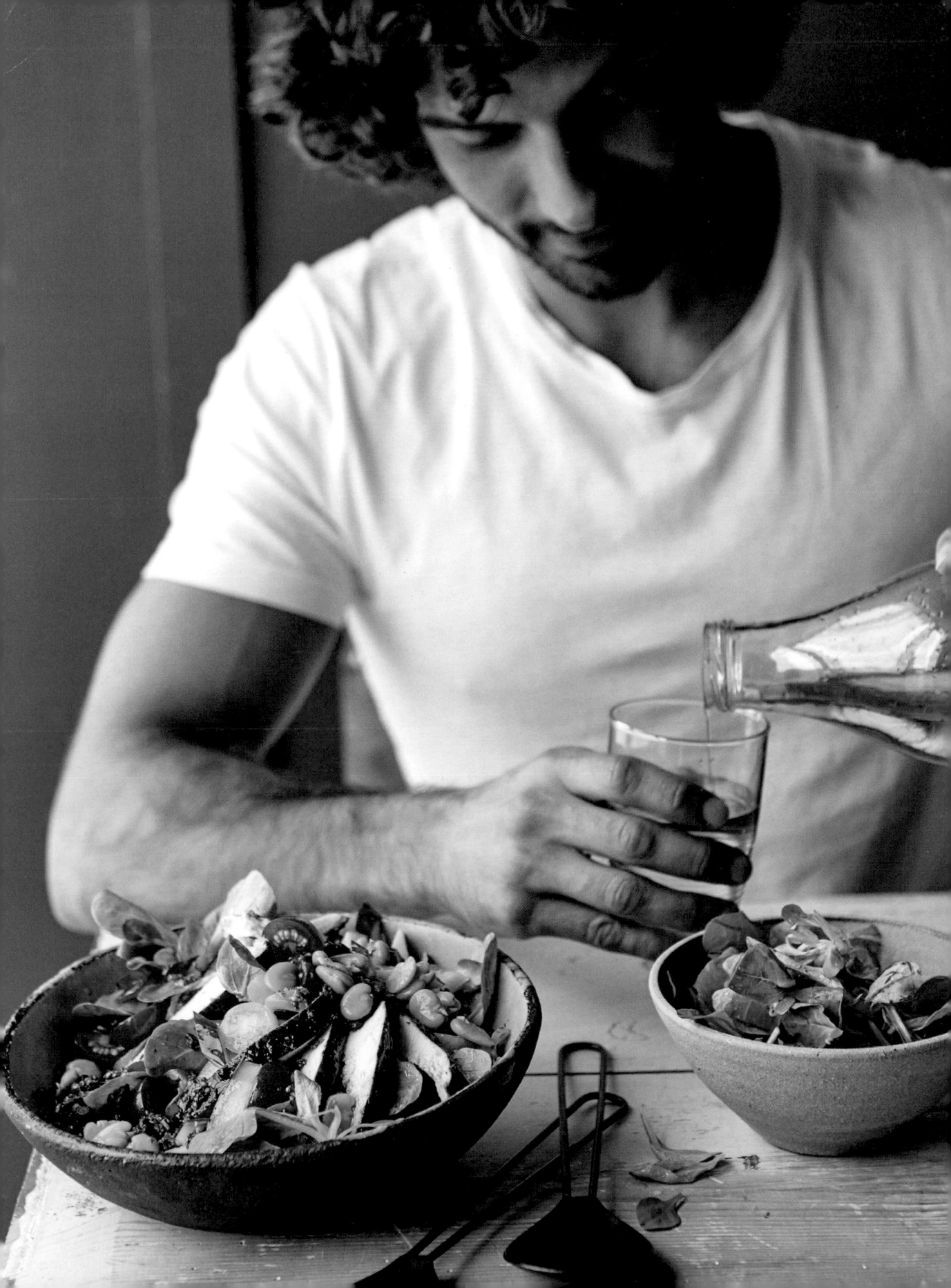

Rosemary and Lemon Chicken with Fennel Slaw

If you've never tried fennel before then this recipe is for you. The fresh and crunchy slaw tastes banging with the chicken.

Ingredients

1 tbsp rosemary leaves, finely chopped
zest and juice of 1 lemon
¼ tsp dried red chilli flakes
salt and pepper
1 x 180–200g skinless chicken breast fillet

For the slaw

1 small fennel bulb, cored, halved and very thinly sliced
50g red cabbage, very finely shredded
50g green cabbage, very finely shredded
2 tbsp finely chopped flat-leaf parsley
1 tbsp dijon mustard
2 tbsp apple cider vinegar

Method

Mix the rosemary, lemon zest and juice and chilli flakes in a bowl.

Make 3–4 deep diagonal slashes on the chicken breast and coat it with the herb and lemon mixture. Season with salt and pepper.

Preheat the grill to medium-high. Place the chicken on a grill rack and place under the grill. Cook for 8–10 minutes, turning halfway through, until the chicken is lightly browned and cooked through. Check by slicing into it to make sure the meat is white all the way through, with no raw pink bits left, then cut it up into thin slices.

Meanwhile, make the slaw by combining all of the ingredients in a bowl. Season and toss to mix well.

Pile the slaw onto a serving plate, top with the chicken and serve.

Reduced-carb

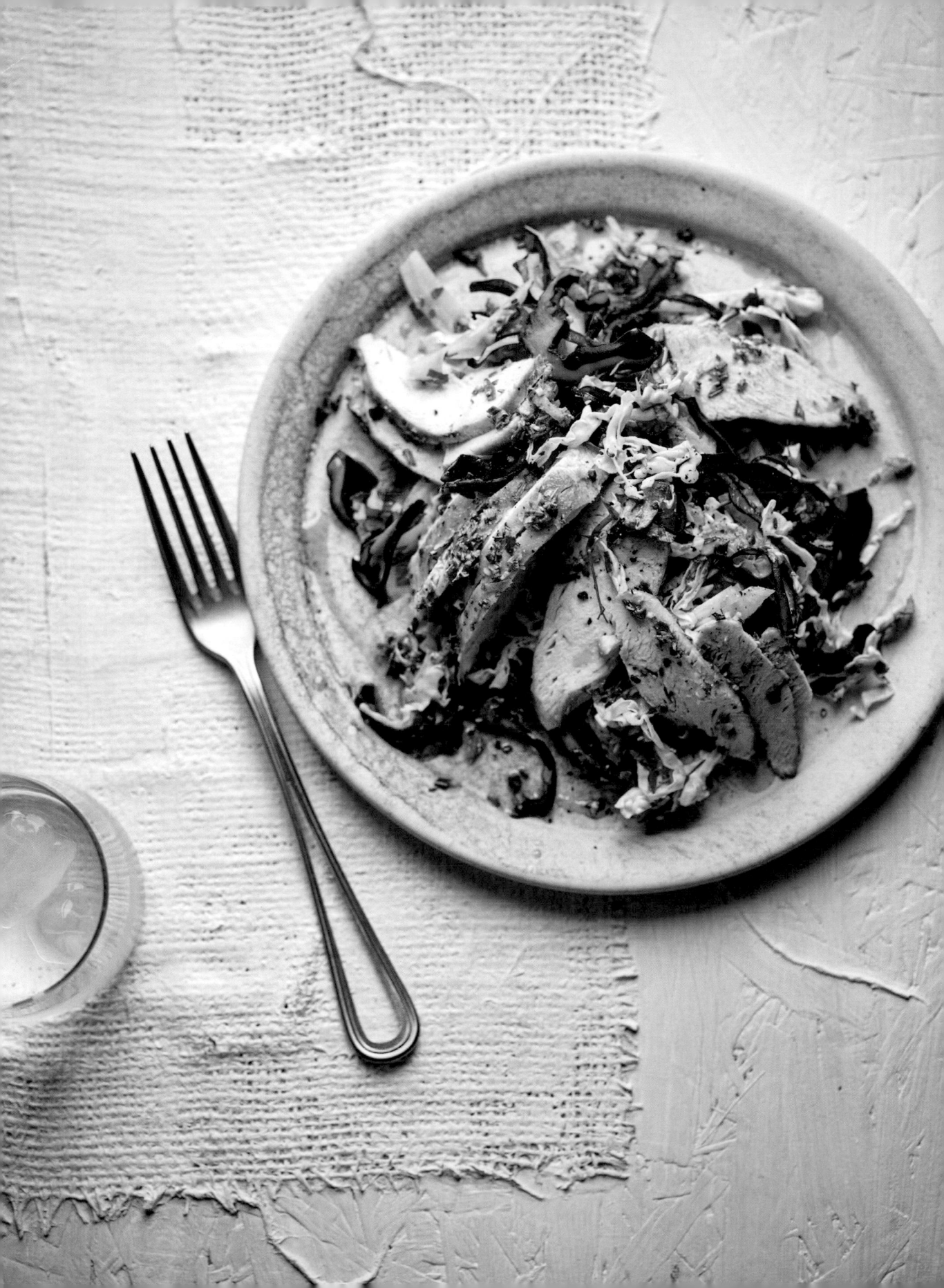

Naked Lamb and Feta Burger with Beetroot Relish

Burgers are without doubt my favourite thing in the world to eat. I've made sure to include at least one good burger recipe in each of my books. This one using lamb and feta tastes incredible.

Ingredients

250g extra-lean lamb mince
1 banana shallot, very finely diced
1 tbsp finely grated orange zest
1 tbsp oregano, finely chopped, or 1 tsp dried oregano
pinch of celery salt
pinch of grated nutmeg
1 tsp finely grated garlic
40g feta cheese, crumbled
2–3 crisp iceberg lettuce leaves, roughly torn
1 ripe plum tomato, sliced
¼ cucumber, sliced

For the beetroot relish

1 cooked beetroot, finely diced or grated
¼ red onion, finely chopped
2 tsp apple cider vinegar
½ tbsp cranberry sauce
½ tbsp wholegrain mustard
salt and pepper

Method

Make the burger by placing the lamb mince in a bowl with the shallot, orange zest, oregano, celery salt, nutmeg, garlic and feta.

Use your hands to mix it all until really well combined. Shape it into a patty and place on a grill rack.

Preheat the grill to medium-high. Slide the burger under the grill and cook for 3–4 minutes on each side, or until cooked through.

Meanwhile, make the beetroot relish by mixing all the ingredients in a bowl. Season with salt and pepper and mix well.

To serve, place the lettuce leaves, sliced tomato and cucumber onto a serving plate. Top with the burger and spoon over the beetroot relish. Enjoy!

Reduced-carb

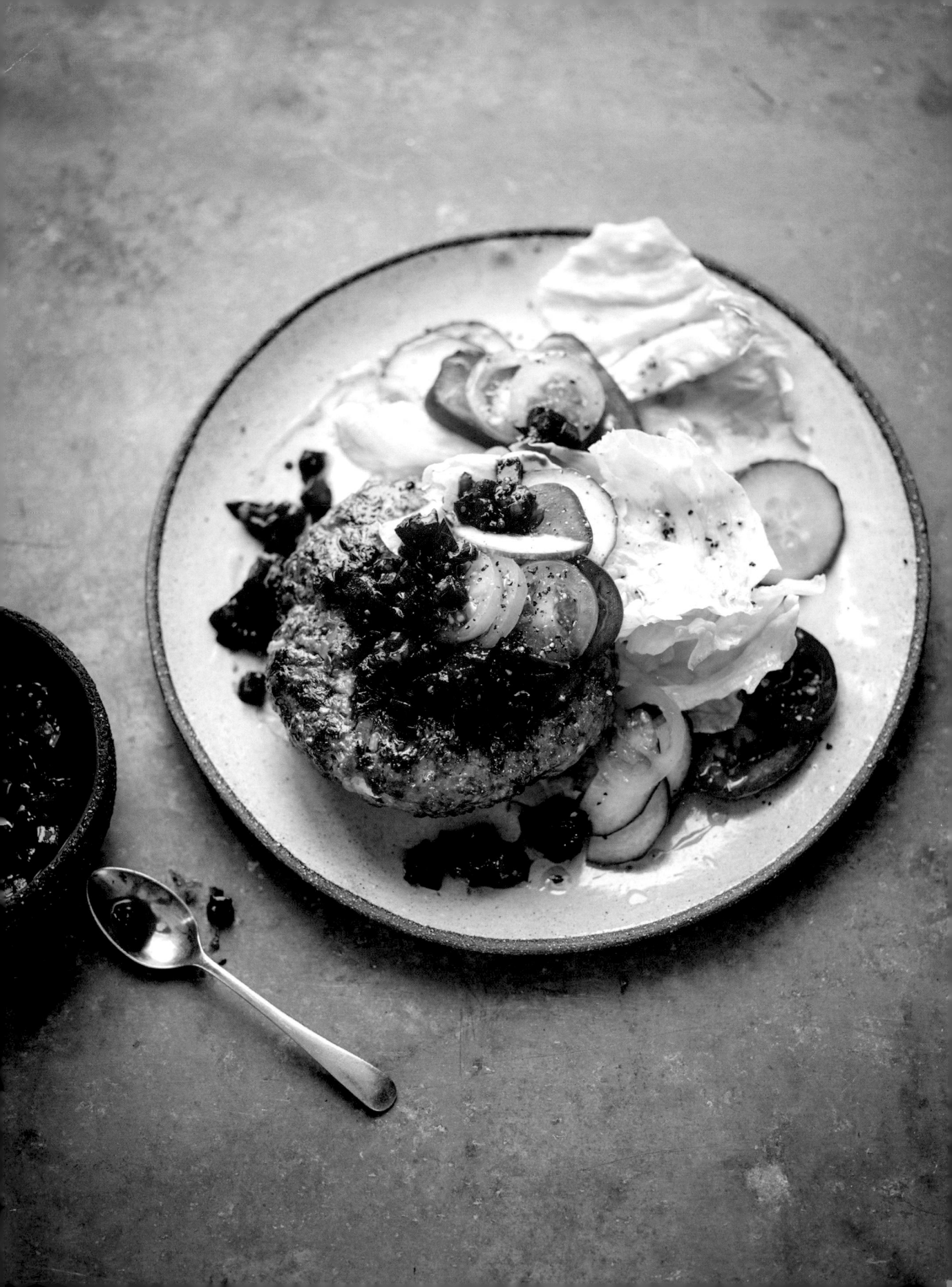

Sweet Chilli Pork and Vegetable Stir-fry

Nothing beats a stir-fry for speed and flavour. When I first began cooking healthy recipes on Instagram, I started with simple meals like this.

Ingredients

1 x 200g lean pork tenderloin
3 tbsp dark soy sauce
2 tbsp mirin
2 tbsp sweet chilli sauce
1 tsp finely grated
   ginger
1 tsp finely grated garlic
1 red chilli, finely chopped
   – remove the seeds if
   you don't like it hot
½ tbsp coconut oil
200g pack mixed stir-fry
   vegetables
1 x 225g tin of sliced bamboo
   shoots, drained
1 x 225g tin of sliced water
   chestnuts, drained
small handful of coriander
   sprigs, for garnish

Method

Cut the pork into thin slices and place in a stainless-steel, ceramic or glass bowl.

Mix together the soy sauce, mirin, sweet chilli sauce, ginger, garlic and chilli and add to the pork. Toss to mix well.

Melt half of the oil in a wide non-stick frying pan and when hot, drain the pork, reserving the marinade. Fry the pork over a medium heat for 4–5 minutes, or until just cooked. Transfer to a plate, cover and keep warm.

Melt the remaining oil in the same pan. Add the vegetables, bamboo shoots and water chestnuts and stir-fry over a medium to high heat for 2–3 minutes, or until piping hot.

Return the pork to the pan with the reserved marinade and continue to stir-fry for 2–3 minutes until piping hot.

Scoop the mixture into a bowl and top with the coriander.

Reduced-carb

Sweet Smoked Paprika Beef Cakes

These come out a bit like mini burgers and taste amazing. Smoked paprika is one of the best flavours to mix with minced beef. Serve it with a nice big mixed-leaf salad.

Ingredients

½ tbsp coconut oil
½ onion, very finely diced
1 portobello mushroom,
 very finely chopped
180g extra-lean beef
 steak mince
2 tbsp flat-leaf parsley,
 finely chopped
1 tsp garlic salt
2 tsp sweet smoked paprika
mixed-leaf salad, to serve

Method

Melt half of the oil in a non-stick frying pan over a medium heat. Add the onion and mushroom and cook for 5 minutes, stirring regularly, until well softened.

Tip into a heatproof bowl and leave to cool for 5 minutes. Add the beef, parsley, garlic salt and sweet smoked paprika. Mix well and shape into three balls. Flatten into patty shapes, each around 2cm thick.

Clean the pan and return to the hob. Heat the remaining oil and cook the 'cakes' over a low to medium heat for 6–8 minutes, turning occasionally, until browned on the outside and cooked through. Serve with the salad.

Reduced-carb

Mexican Beef with Lime and Avocado Salsa

OMG look at that photo. How tasty does that look? If you love Mexican food then this recipe is a dream come true.

Ingredients

1 x 200g beef minute steak
1 red pepper
1–2 tbsp Mexican spice mix
  (or Cajun)
½ tbsp coconut oil
1 tbsp soured cream (optional)
½ lime, cut into slices,
  to serve
big green salad, to serve

For the salsa

1 avocado, de-stoned and
  cut into 1cm dice
2 ripe plum tomatoes, cut
  into 1cm dice
1 red chilli, finely chopped
½ red onion, finely diced
juice of 2 limes
small handful of chopped
  coriander, plus extra for
  garnish
1 tbsp toasted pine nuts
salt and pepper

Method

Throw all of the salsa ingredients into a bowl. Season with salt and black pepper and set aside.

Thinly slice the beef steak and pepper and place in a bowl with the spice mix. Toss to mix well.

Melt the oil in a wide non-stick frying pan. Place the beef and pepper in the pan and stir-fry for 1–2 minutes over a high heat until browned and cooked through.

Serve on a plate with the salsa and soured cream, if using. Top with the coriander sprigs and slices of lime, and serve with the big green salad.

Reduced-carb

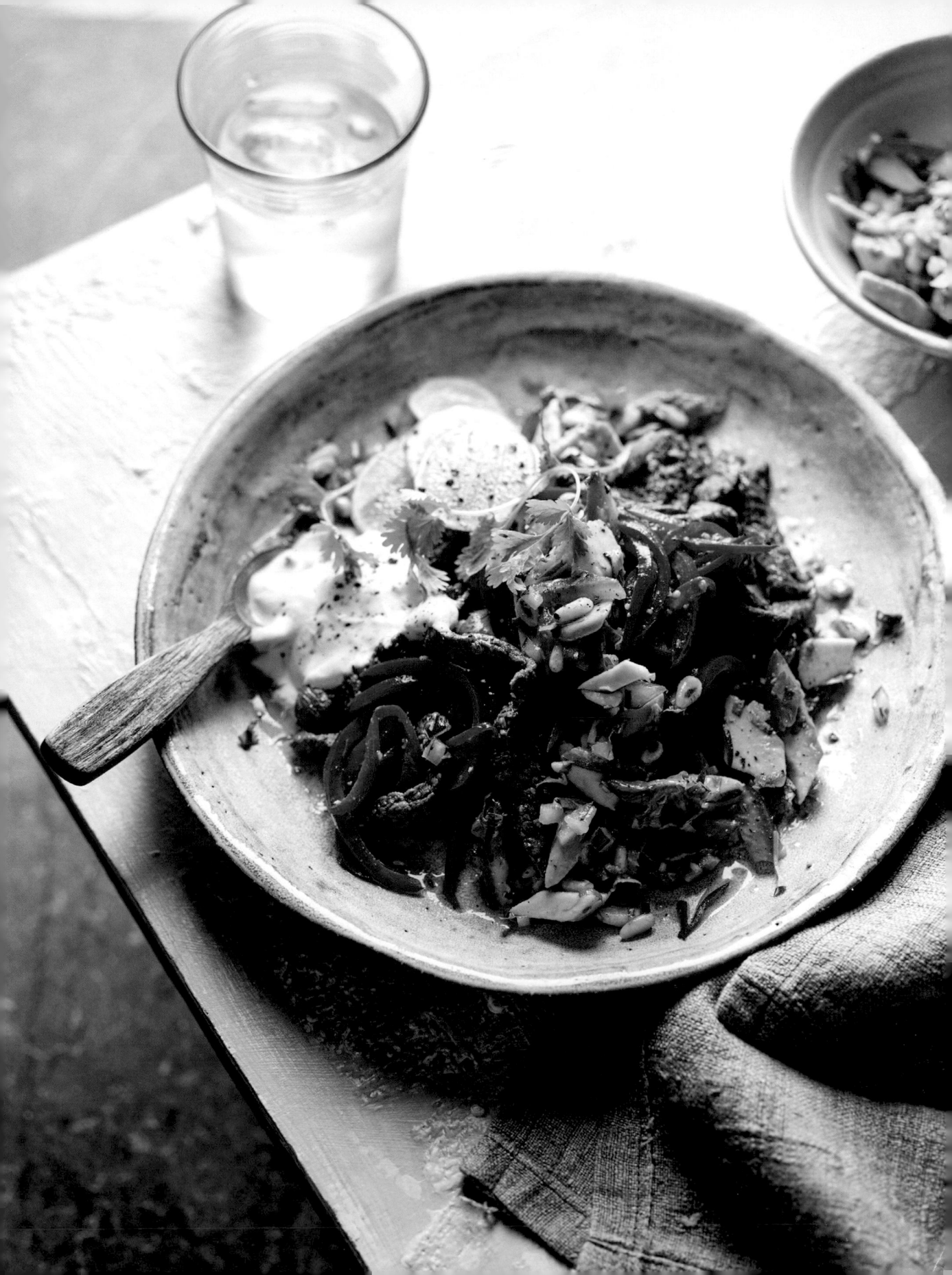

Sweet Chilli Fish and Vegetable Skewers

It's great to get some fish into your diet and this recipe is super easy and tasty. Serve it with half a mashed avocado or a dollop of Greek yoghurt.

Ingredients

1 clove garlic, crushed
½ tbsp sweet chilli sauce
2 tbsp light soy sauce
½ tbsp apple cider vinegar
1 tbsp very finely chopped
  spring onion (green part only)
1 x 200g skinless white fish
  fillet, such as cod, halibut
  or monkfish
2 baby courgettes, each cut
  into four pieces
6 cherry tomatoes
50g mixed baby leaf salad
juice of ½ lemon
salt and pepper

Method

Place the garlic, sweet chilli sauce, soy sauce, vinegar and spring onion in a wide stainless-steel, ceramic or glass bowl.

Cut the fish fillet into 6–8 even-sized chunks and place them in the garlic marinade. Toss to mix well.

When you're ready to cook, thread the fish onto two metal skewers, alternating with the pieces of courgette and cherry tomatoes. Place them on the grill rack.

Preheat the grill to medium-high.

Brush the skewers with with the leftover marinade and slide them under the grill, making sure the grill rack is about 10cm away from the heat to ensure even cooking. Allow to cook for 6–8 minutes, turning halfway through, until the fish is cooked and the vegetables are tender.

Chuck the salad leaves on a plate and squeeze over the lemon juice. Season well, top with the skewers and enjoy.

Reduced-carb

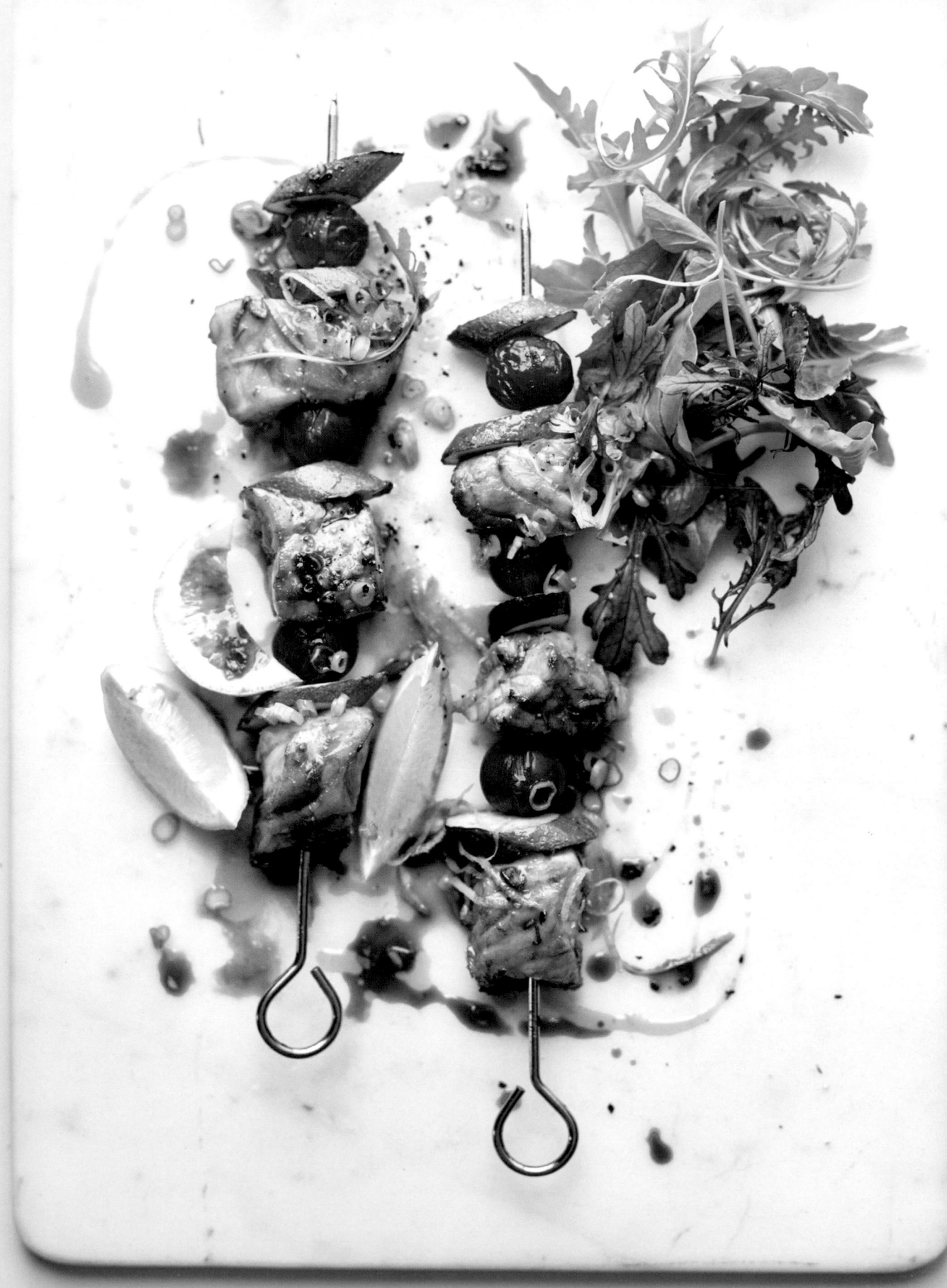

Crispy Cod with Teriyaki and Sesame Stir-fry

This is my favourite photo in this whole book. I just want to eat it off the page. The teriyaki flavours in this recipe help it to taste as good as it looks.

Ingredients

2 tbsp teriyaki sauce
1 tbsp sweet chilli sauce
zest and juice of 1 lime
1 x 180–190g cod fillet, skin-on
½ tbsp coconut oil
300g pack stir-fry vegetables
2 tbsp soy sauce
1 tbsp toasted sesame seeds

Method

Mix the teriyaki sauce, sweet chilli sauce and the lime zest and juice in a large bowl. Add the cod fillet and turn to coat evenly.

Melt the coconut oil in a non-stick frying pan over a medium heat. Reserving the marinade, drain the fish and fry skin-side down, for 4–5 minutes, until slightly crisp and blackened.

Turn over the fish and cook for another 2–3 minutes, or until cooked through. Set aside.

Cook the stir-fry vegetables in another pan with a splash of water and add the soy sauce and reserved marinade, cooking for a further 2–3 minutes or according to the packet instructions.

Pile the stir-fry vegetables onto a plate and top with the crispy cod. Scatter over the sesame seeds and serve.

Reduced-carb

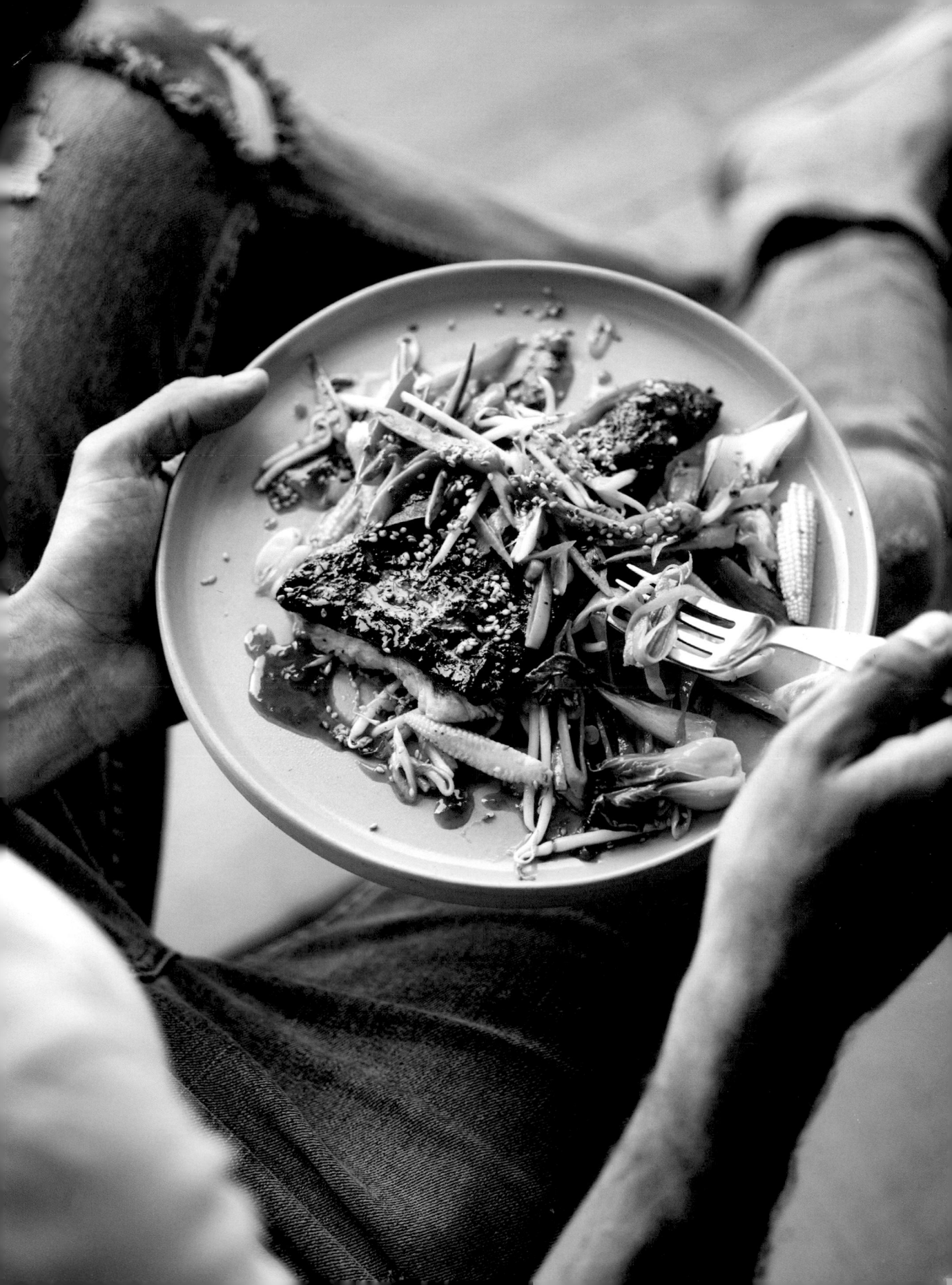

Grilled Italian Mackerel with Chunky Salsa Verde

Here's a recipe full of those essential omega-3 fatty acids. The salsa verde brings so much flavour to this dish.

Ingredients

1 each red and yellow peppers,
  de-seeded and cut into
  thin strips
½ onion, thinly sliced
2 x 100g mackerel fillets,
  skin-on
salt and pepper
small handful of wild rocket

For the salsa verde

3 tbsp basil leaves, chopped
1 tbsp tarragon leaves, chopped
  (optional)
1 tbsp mint leaves, chopped
3 tbsp flat-leaf parsley, chopped
1 clove garlic, crushed
1 anchovy fillet in oil, drained
1 tsp capers, rinsed and drained
¼ tsp dried red chilli flakes
juice of ½ lemon
50ml cooled vegetable stock
½ tbsp extra-virgin olive oil

Method

Place all the salsa verde ingredients in a small food processor and blitz until well combined. You might need to add an extra splash of stock to get it all moving. Set aside.

Heat a large, ridged non-stick griddle pan until hot and add the peppers and onions. Cook for 6–8 minutes, turning frequently until softened and char-grilled.

Preheat the grill to high. While the peppers are cooking, score the mackerel skin diagonally with a sharp knife, and place on a grill rack, skin-side up. Season with salt and pepper. Place under the grill and cook for 5–6 minutes, or until cooked through.

Toss the griddled peppers and onions with the rocket and place on a serving plate.

Top with the mackerel and spoon over the salsa verde before serving.

Chicken, Bacon and Quinoa Salad with Halloumi Cheese

This literally contains all of my favourite ingredients in one bowl. If you haven't tried halloumi cheese yet you are going to love it.

Ingredients

1 x 180g skinless chicken breast fillet
¾ tbsp coconut oil
1 lean rasher of bacon (all visible fat removed)
50g midget trees (tenderstem broccoli), thinly sliced
100g pre-cooked red and white quinoa
1 jarred red pepper, drained and chopped
1 tbsp coriander, finely chopped
1 ripe avocado, de-stoned, and roughly chopped
2 spring onions, finely sliced
1 tbsp preserved lemon, finely chopped (optional)
1 tbsp apple cider vinegar
pinch of ground cinnamon
juice of ½ orange
salt and pepper
30g slice of halloumi cheese (about 1cm thick)

Method

Place the chicken between two pieces of cling film, and using a rolling pin or wooden mallet, lightly beat until slightly thinned to an even thickness.

Melt ½ tablespoon of the coconut oil on a hot griddle pan and cook the chicken for 6–8 minutes on each side, until cooked through. Check by slicing into it to make sure the meat is white all the way through, with no raw pink bits left.

Meanwhile, preheat the grill to high. Cook the bacon rasher under the grill for 2–3 minutes until crispy. Drain on kitchen roll, then cut into strips with kitchen scissors. Set aside.

In a small saucepan of lightly salted boiling water, blanch the broccoli for 2 minutes. Drain and place in a wide bowl with the cooked quinoa and roasted red pepper.

Roughly shred the chicken and add to the quinoa mixture with the chopped coriander, avocado, spring onions and preserved lemon, if using.

Stir in the apple cider vinegar, cinnamon and orange juice, season and toss to mix well.

Melt the remaining coconut oil in a small frying pan and add the halloumi. Cook for 1–2 minutes on each side, or until golden. Remove and roughly chop.

Place the salad in a bowl, scatter over the halloumi and bacon and get stuck in.

Reduced-carb

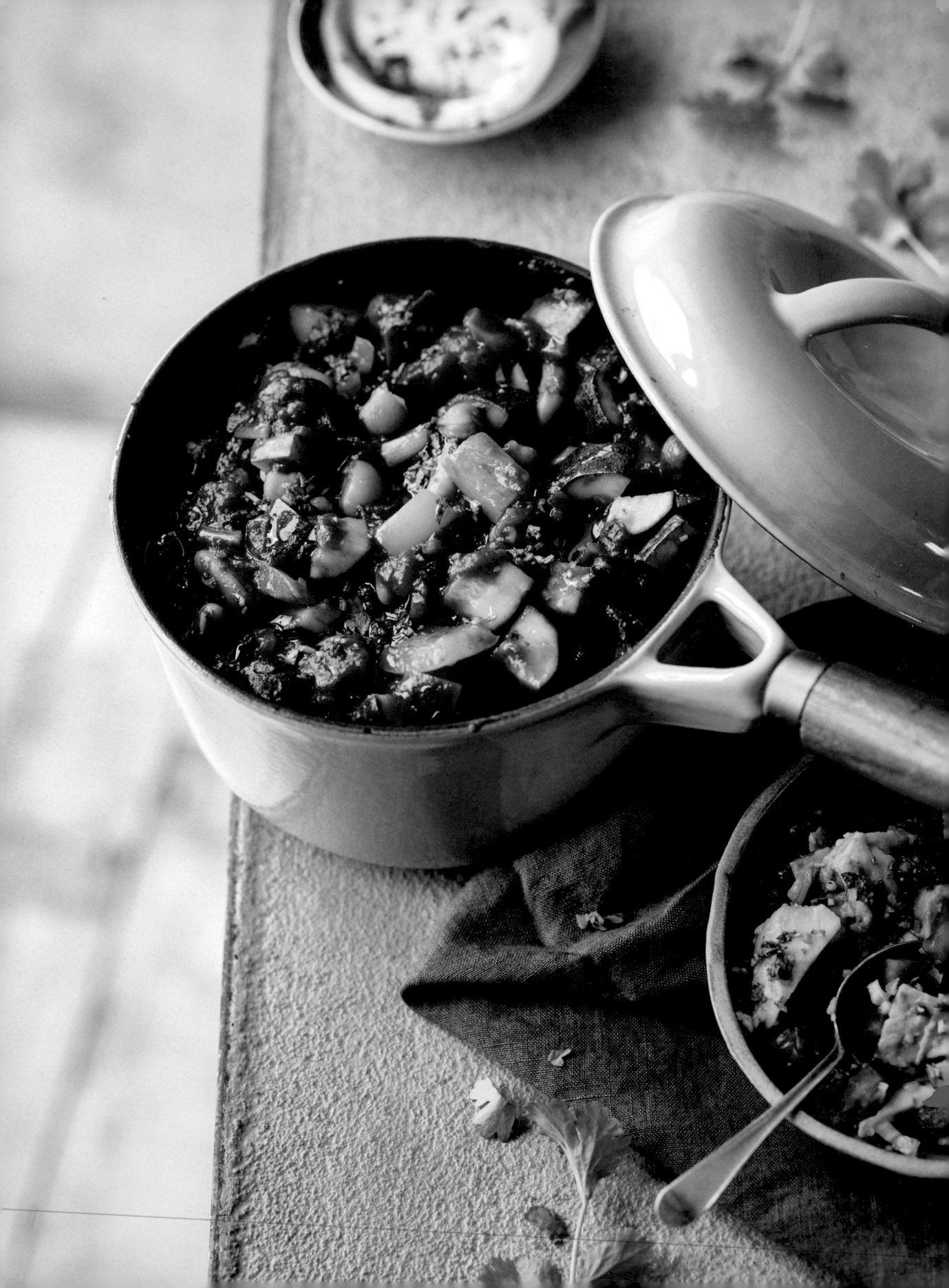

Veggie Mixed Bean Chilli with Guacamole

Serves
1

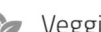 Veggie
⏱ Make ahead

Here's a great recipe for those days when you don't fancy eating meat and want a veggie option. I've got some good news, too … I've decided my seventh book will be a vegetarian cookbook!

Ingredients

1 tbsp coconut oil
½ small red onion, finely diced
½ yellow pepper, de-seeded and finely diced
½ courgette, finely diced
3 tsp Cajun spice mix
½ tsp ground cumin
¼ tsp ground cinnamon
½ x 400g tin of chopped tomatoes
4 tbsp tomato puree
75ml vegetable stock
1 x 400g tin of mixed pulses and beans in water, drained
salt and pepper
1 tbsp soured cream

For the guacamole

1 avocado, de-stoned and cut into 1cm dice
1 shallot, finely diced
1 clove garlic, crushed
1 ripe plum tomato, finely chopped
juice of 1 large lime
small handful of chopped coriander (leaves and stalks), plus extra for garnish

Method

Melt the oil in a wide non-stick frying pan over a high heat. Add the onion, pepper, courgette, Cajun spice mix, cumin and cinnamon and stir-fry for 2–3 minutes.

Add the tomatoes, puree, stock and the tin of mixed pulses and beans and bring to the boil. Cook over a medium to high heat for 6–8 minutes, or until thickened. Season well and remove from the heat.

Meanwhile, make the guacamole by mixing all the ingredients in a bowl. Season well.

Spoon the chilli into a wide bowl and top with the soured cream. Serve with the guacamole, topped with extra coriander.

Reduced-carb

Grilled Sea Bass with Chilli and Ginger

Don't be scared to get the fish skin really crispy. It makes it taste amazing. You'll be coming back to make this again, I'm sure.

Ingredients

2 x 100g sea bass fillets, skin-on
salt and pepper
1 tbsp coconut oil
2cm piece of ginger, peeled and shredded into very thin matchsticks
1 clove garlic, very thinly sliced
1 long red chilli, de-seeded and very thinly shredded
4 spring onions, shredded lengthways
1 tbsp dark soy sauce
1 tsp mirin
steamed greens, to serve

Method

Season the fish with salt and pepper, then slash the skin diagonally three times with a short, sharp knife. Preheat the grill to medium-high.

Place the fish on a grill rack, skin-side up. Place under the grill for 6–8 minutes, or until lightly charred at the edges and cooked through. Transfer to a plate and keep warm.

Melt the oil in a small non-stick frying pan, then fry the ginger, garlic and chilli over a gentle heat for about 2 minutes until golden.

Remove the pan from the heat and toss in the spring onions. Splash the fish with the soy sauce and mirin and spoon over the contents of the pan. Serve with steamed greens of your choice.

Reduced-carb

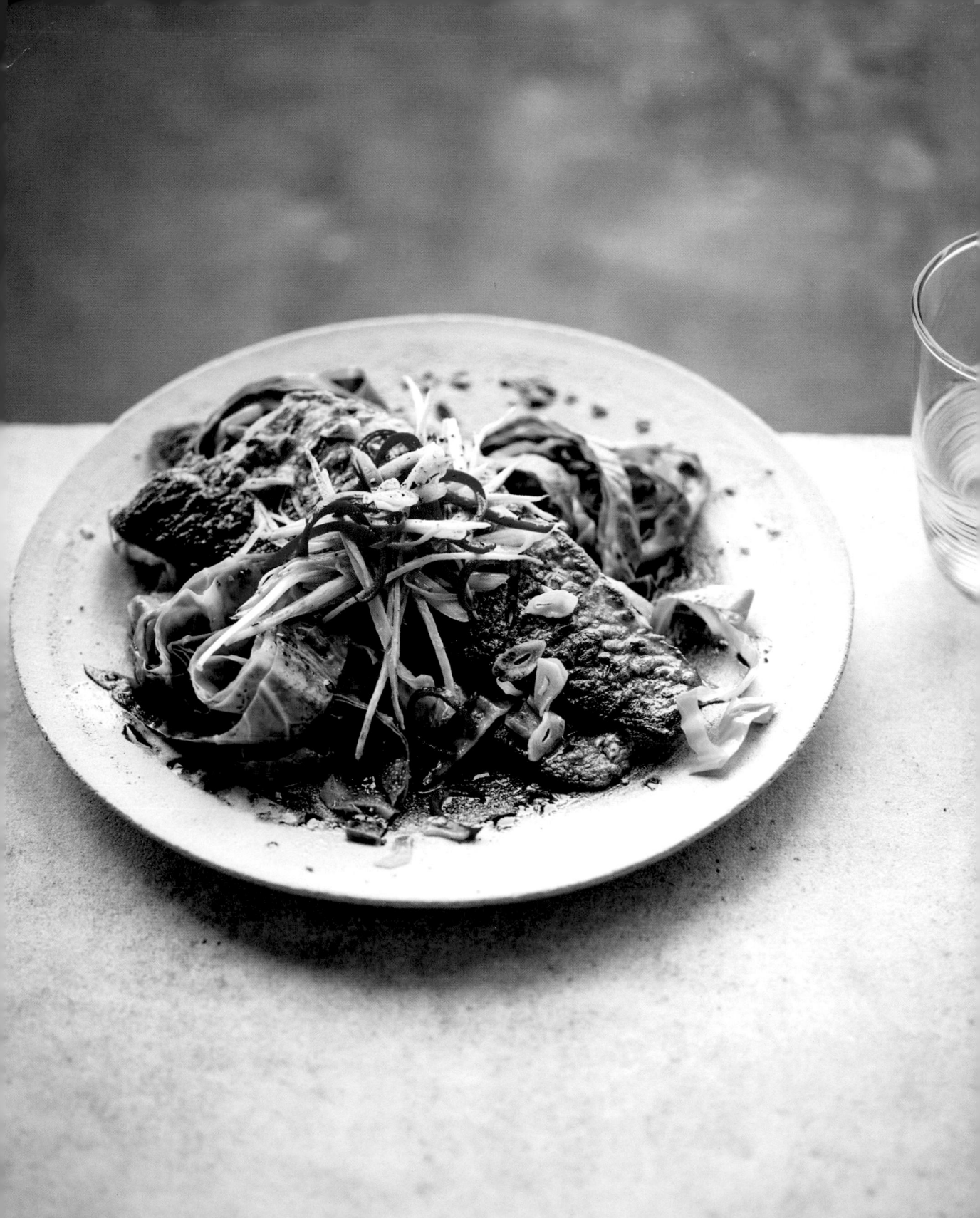

Italian Chicken Sausage Ragu with a Fried Egg

It may seem like an odd combo to mix chicken sausages with soya beans but it tastes absolutely amazing and is really filling. Do yourself a favour and give this a try. I promise you will love it.

Ingredients

3–4 chicken sausages
  (around 250g)
1 tbsp coconut oil
1 tsp fennel seeds
¼ tsp dried chilli flakes
3 tbsp tomato puree
200ml chicken stock
200g frozen soya beans
4 tbsp basil leaves
salt and pepper
1 large egg
1–2 tbsp grated pecorino
  cheese to serve

Method

Remove the sausage meat from the casings and set it aside.

Melt half of the oil in a wide non-stick frying pan over a medium heat and fry the fennel seeds and chilli flakes for 1 minute.

Add the sausage meat and stir-fry over a high heat until just brown.

Stir in the tomato puree and stock. Stir to combine, bring to the boil and cook for a further 6–8 minutes until the sauce has reduced and thickened.

Add the soya beans and continue to cook for 2–3 minutes until the sauce is thick and the soya beans are hot and tender.

Remove the pan from the heat and stir in the basil. Season well and spoon into a shallow serving bowl.

Melt the remaining oil in a small non-stick frying pan and crack in the egg. Fry the egg until crispy and cooked through.

Top the ragu with the egg, scatter with the grated pecorino cheese and serve.

Reduced-carb

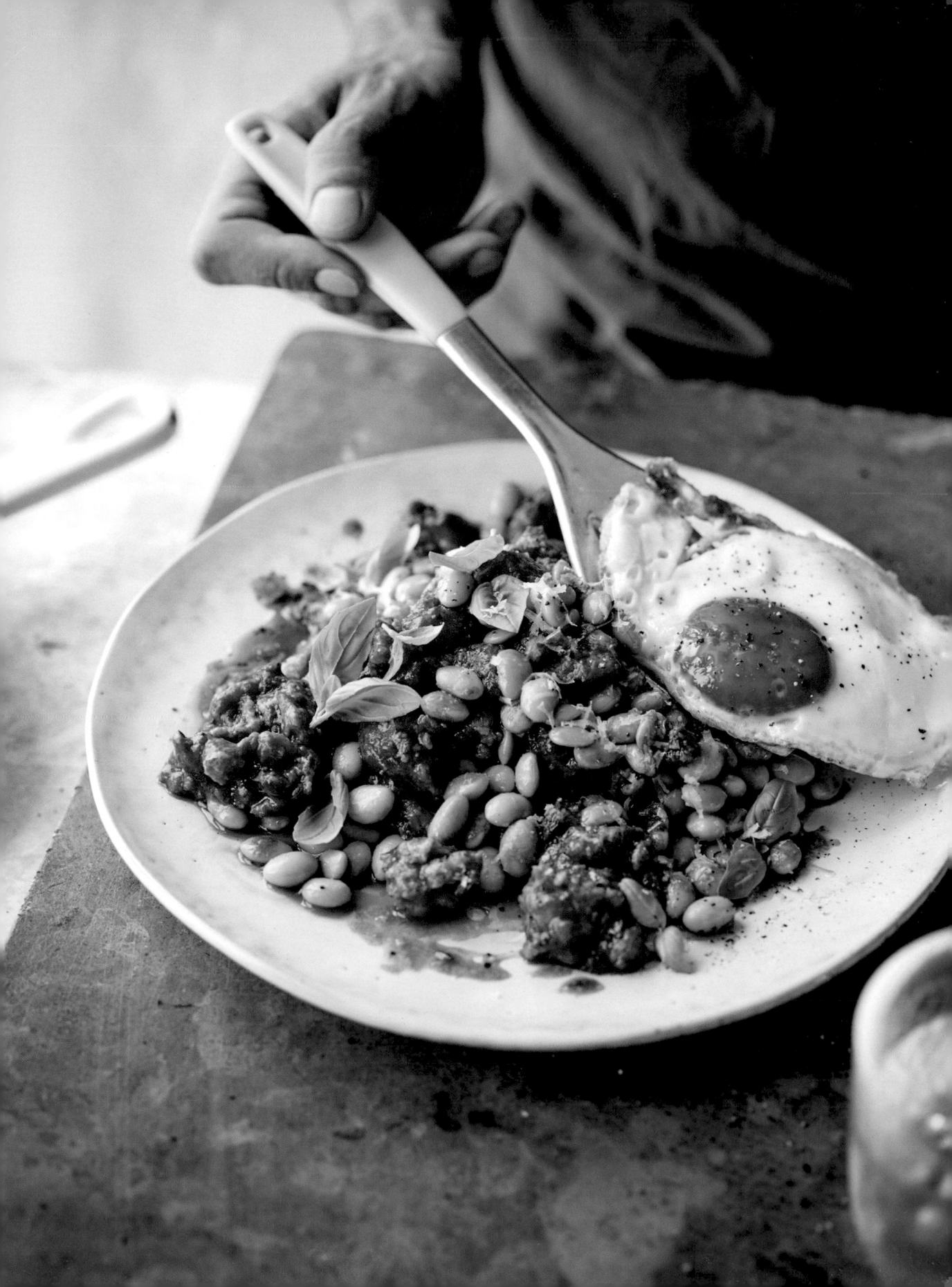

🕐 Make ahead

Mango, Chicken and Avocado Salad

This is a really great salad that you can prep for work the following day. To stop your avocado going brown just leave it whole and cut it open when you get to work.

Ingredients

1 x 180g skinless chicken breast fillet
½ tbsp coconut oil
1 ripe mango, peeled, de-stoned and cut into 1cm slices
2 spring onions, very finely chopped
1 long red chilli, de-seeded and very finely sliced
1 avocado, de-stoned and cut into 1cm pieces
juice of 1 lime, plus extra slices to serve
salt and pepper
small handful of coriander, finely chopped
½ tbsp olive oil
few drops of toasted sesame oil (optional)
1 baby gem lettuce

Method

Place the chicken between two pieces of cling film, and using a rolling pin or wooden mallet, lightly beat until slightly thinned with an even thickness.

Melt ½ tablespoon of coconut oil on a hot griddle pan and cook the chicken for 6–8 minutes on each side, until cooked through. Check by slicing into it to make sure the meat is white all the way through, with no raw pink bits left.

Place the mango (and its juices) in a bowl.

Chuck in the spring onions, chilli and avocado pieces. Stir in the lime juice, season well and toss to combine.

Chop the chicken breast into 1cm pieces and add them to the bowl with the chopped coriander.

Drizzle over the olive oil, toss to mix well and add the sesame oil, if using.

Separate the leaves from the lettuce and add to your plate. Pile on the salad mixture, top with the slices of lime and get stuck in.

Reduced-carb

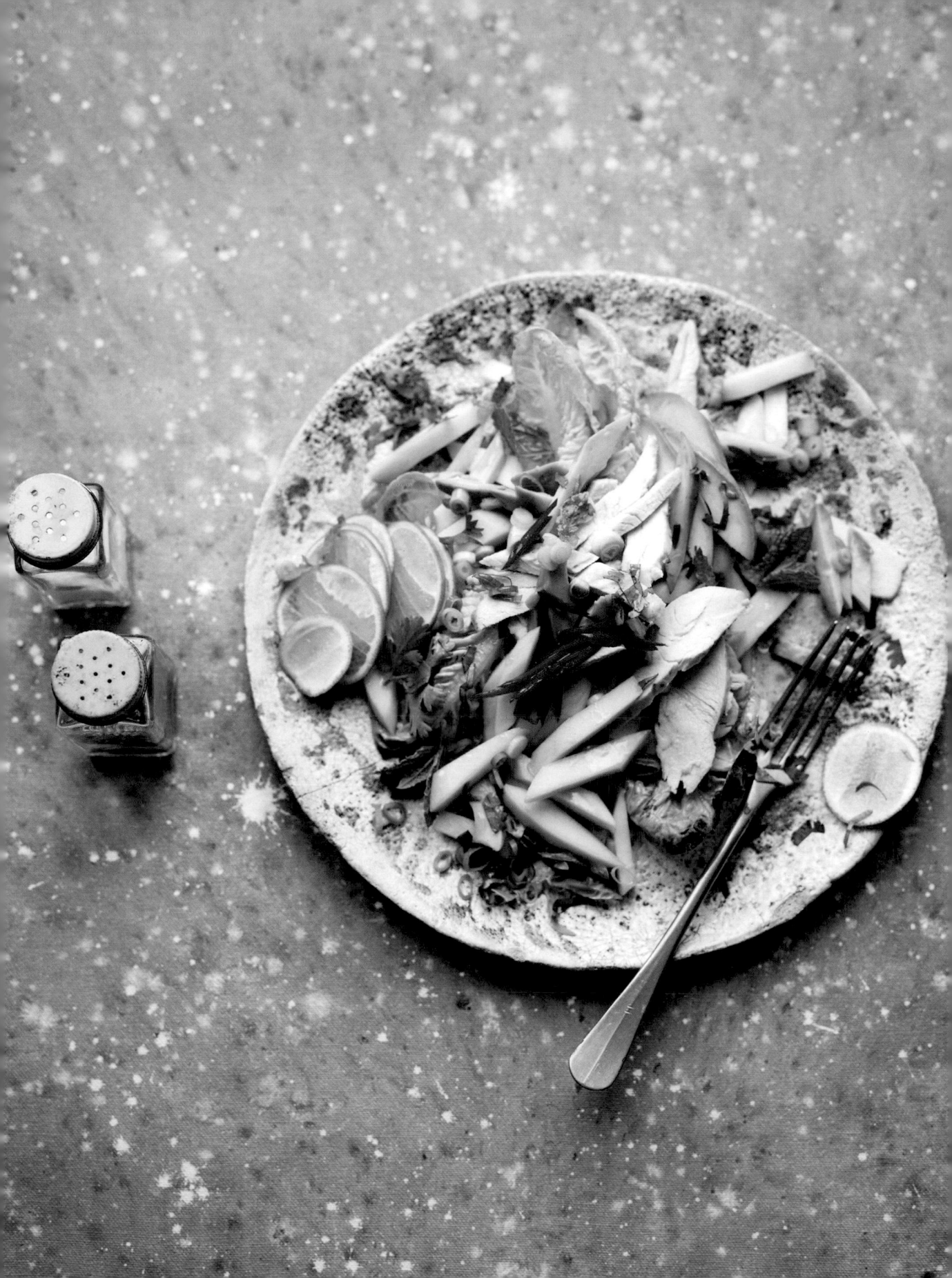

Joe's Cheesy Meatball Skewers

Meatballs and grilled cheese. What more could you want? You could also throw this recipe on the barbecue.

Ingredients

250g extra-lean steak mince
salt and pepper
1 red pepper, de-seeded and cut into bite-sized pieces
1 yellow pepper, de-seeded and cut into bite-sized pieces
4 cherry tomatoes
1 small red onion, peeled and cut into 8 wedges
2 tbsp grated cheddar cheese
big green salad, to serve

For the herby yoghurt drizzle

½ clove garlic, crushed
100ml natural yoghurt
juice of ½ lemon
3 tbsp parsley, very finely chopped

Method

Mix the steak mince with salt and pepper and knead until well combined. Shape into six meatballs. Preheat the grill to medium-high.

Whisk together all the ingredients for the herby yoghurt drizzle.

Alternating between each ingredient, thread the meatballs, peppers, cherry tomatoes and red onion pieces onto two metal skewers. Place them on a grill rack under the grill and cook for 5–6 minutes.

Turn the skewers over, scatter the cheese over the meatballs and grill for a further 5–6 minutes, or until lightly golden and cooked through.

Place on a serving plate with the salad and drizzle over the herby yoghurt.

Reduced-carb

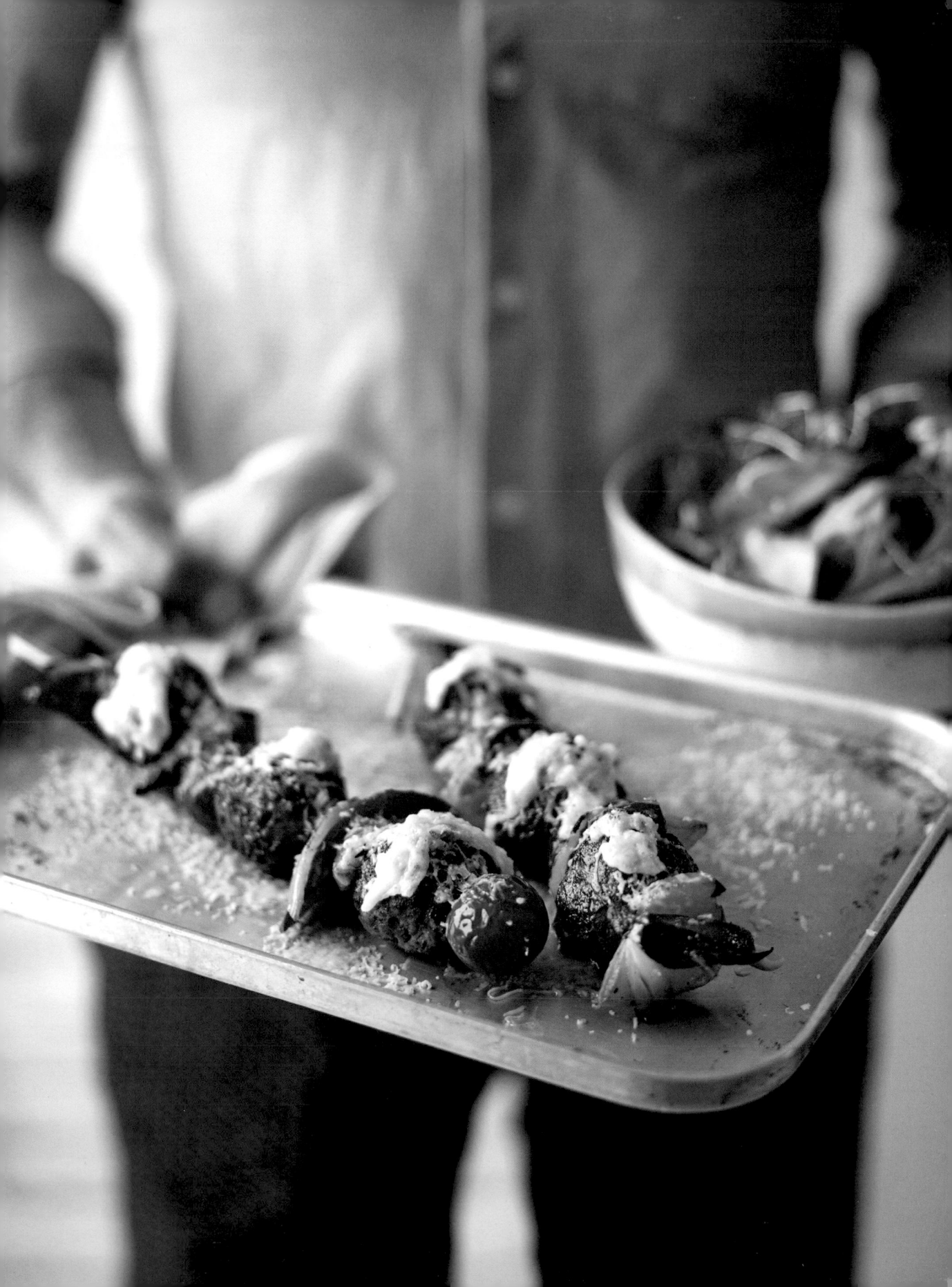

Chicken Escalope with Roasted Courgette

This is such a simple recipe to make and full of flavour. This will taste good at lunch, dinner or even breakfast!

Ingredients

½ courgette, cut into 1cm dice
½ red pepper, de-seeded and
  cut into 1cm pieces
½ yellow pepper, de-seeded
  and cut into bite-sized pieces
½ red onion, cut into
  1cm pieces
2 tbsp balsamic vinegar
1 tsp dried oregano
salt and pepper
1 x 180–200g skinless chicken
  breast fillet
1 tbsp olive oil
1 large clove garlic, crushed
1 tsp finely chopped thyme
  leaves
zest and juice of ½ lemon
1–2 tbsp flat-leaf parsley,
  finely chopped

Method

Preheat the oven to 220°C (fan 200°C/gas mark 7).

Line a large roasting tray with non-stick baking parchment. Place the vegetables in the tray and drizzle with the balsamic. Scatter over the oregano, season well and cook in the oven for 12–15 minutes, or until tender.

Meanwhile, place the chicken between two sheets of cling film and bash with a rolling pin until it is about 1cm thick.

Place the oil in a small bowl with the garlic, thyme, lemon zest and juice. Mix well, then spread over the chicken.

Heat a non-stick, ridged griddle pan until smoking and add the chicken. Cook for 3–4 minutes on each side, or until completely cooked through. Check by slicing into it to make sure the meat is white all the way through, with no raw pink bits left.

To serve, spoon the vegetables and any pan juices onto a plate and top with the chicken. Scatter the parsley over the top and serve.

One-Pan Caprese Fish

This recipe uses melted mozzarella cheese, fresh basil and balsamic vinegar, meaning it tastes like a dream. Enjoy.

Ingredients

1 tbsp coconut oil
1 small onion, finely diced
2 cloves garlic, crushed
1 x 400g tin of chopped tomatoes (or 3–4 fresh tomatoes, roughly chopped)
salt and pepper
1 tbsp balsamic vinegar
large handful of baby spinach leaves
1 x 180–200g skinless cod fillet
1 slice of mozzarella (about 20–30g)
2 tbsp basil leaves, finely chopped

Method

Melt the oil in a medium non-stick frying pan and add the onion, garlic and chopped tomatoes. Season well and bring to the boil over a high heat.

Add the balsamic and allow to cook for 4–5 minutes. Chuck in the spinach and stir to combine.

Season the cod and place it on top of the tomato mixture. Top with the mozzarella and basil.

Cover and cook over a medium heat for 8–10 minutes or until the fish is cooked through and the cheese has just melted. Season to taste and eat straight from the pan.

Chicken Saltimbocca with Spinach

This is an absolute classic. Everyone in the family will love this one. I like doubling the recipe and making this when my friends come over for dinner.

Ingredients

1 x 180–200g skinless
  chicken breast fillet
salt and pepper
1 tsp dried sage
1 tbsp coconut oil
300g red or yellow cherry
  tomatoes, halved
30g baby spinach leaves
2 cloves garlic, finely chopped
1–2 slices parma ham
30g pizza mozzarella cheese,
  grated
1 tbsp flat-leaf parsley,
  finely chopped

Method

Place the chicken between two pieces of cling film, and using a rolling pin or wooden mallet, lightly beat until about 1cm thick. Season well and sprinkle over the sage.

Melt half of the oil in a non-stick frying pan. Add the chicken and cook for 2–3 minutes. Flip the chicken and continue searing until the other side is browned and the chicken is cooked through, about 2–3 minutes. Check by slicing into it to make sure the meat is white all the way through, with no raw pink bits left. Transfer the chicken to a plate and cover with tin foil.

Lower the heat to medium and melt the remaining oil. Add the tomatoes, season well, and stir-fry for 1–2 minutes. Stir in the spinach and garlic and cook until just wilted, about 2 minutes. Remove the frying pan from the heat.

Preheat the grill to high. Place the chicken on top of the vegetables. Scrunch the parma ham over the top of the chicken, then sprinkle over the cheese.

Place the pan under the grill and cook for 45–50 seconds, until the cheese is melted and bubbling. Serve topped with the chopped parsley.

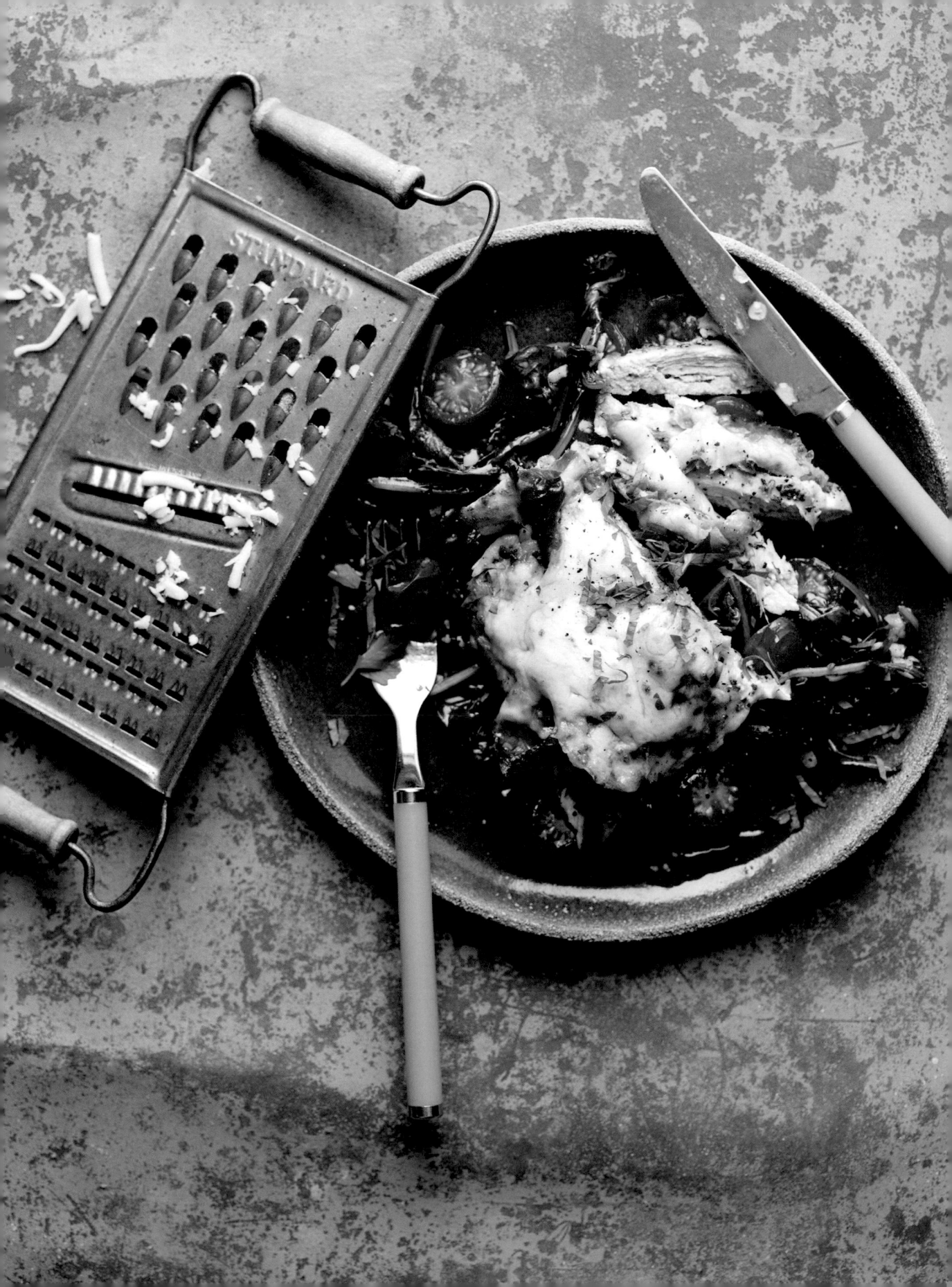

Charred Sprout and Chicken Salad

I used to think boiled Brussels sprouts were awful, smelly things. I wouldn't go near them as a kid but since I've discovered how they transform when you char them over a high heat, I can't get enough of them. They take on a whole new texture and flavour that I love.

Ingredients

1 x 200g skinless chicken breast fillet
1 tbsp coconut oil
150g Brussels sprouts, roughly shredded
1 tsp cumin seeds
1 small red onion, very finely diced
1 medium carrot, coarsely grated
small handful of coriander leaves, roughly chopped
2 tbsp pomegranate seeds (optional)
2 tbsp toasted walnuts, roughly chopped

For the dressing

finely grated zest and juice of 1 large orange
1 tbsp apple cider vinegar
1 tbsp olive oil
1 tsp finely grated ginger
1 tbsp wholegrain mustard
salt and pepper

Method

Place the chicken between two pieces of cling film, and using a rolling pin or wooden mallet, lightly beat until slightly thinned to an even thickness.

Melt ½ tablespoon of the coconut oil on a hot griddle pan and cook the chicken for 6–8 minutes on each side, until cooked through. Check by slicing into it to make sure the meat is white all the way through, with no raw pink bits left.

Melt the remaining oil in a wide non-stick frying pan over a high heat. When it is piping hot, add the sprouts and stir-fry for 8–10 minutes, or until lightly charred and caramelised all over. Set aside.

Toast the cumin seeds in a dry medium-sized non-stick frying pan over a medium heat until fragrant. Remove from the heat.

Whisk all the dressing ingredients into the pan with the cumin seeds. Season well, add the red onion and set aside.

Pile the cooked sprouts on a plate, pour over the dressing and toss to mix well.

Roughly tear the chicken into bite-sized pieces and add to the plate with the carrot, coriander, pomegranate seeds (if using) and walnuts.

Reduced-carb

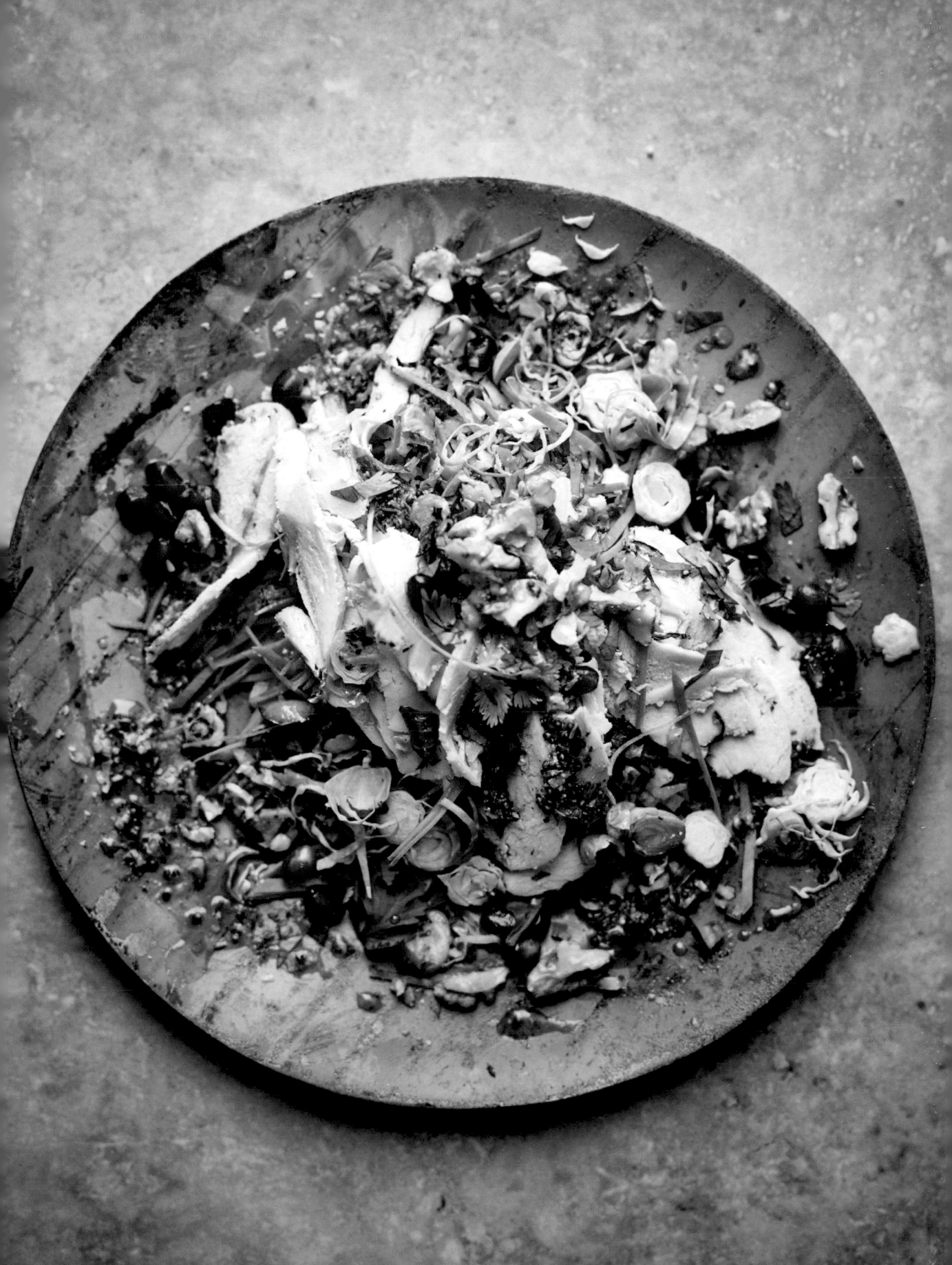

Spicy Chipotle Chicken Bowl with Chunky Guacamole

Homemade guacamole is literally the best thing ever and when you combine it with this tasty chipotle chicken you'll be in food heaven.

Ingredients

250g skinless, boneless chicken thighs, cut into large, bite-sized pieces
1 tbsp chipotle paste
juice of 1 lime, plus extra wedges to serve
salt and pepper
½ tbsp coconut oil
2 red peppers, de-seeded and cut into bite-sized pieces
large dollop of soured cream
1 tbsp grated cheddar cheese
paprika, for sprinkling

For the guacamole

1 avocado, de-stoned and roughly chopped
1 tomato, de-seeded and finely chopped
¼ red onion, finely chopped
2 tbsp coriander, chopped, plus extra for garnish
juice of 1 large lime
1 red chilli, de-seeded and finely diced

Method

Preheat the grill to medium.

Chuck the chicken in a bowl with the chipotle paste and lime juice and season well. Toss to coat evenly, then place the chicken under the grill.

Cook for 5–6 minutes on each side, or until cooked through. Check by slicing into one of the pieces to make sure the meat is white all the way through, with no raw pink bits left.

Meanwhile, melt the oil in a large non-stick frying pan. Add the peppers and cook over a high heat for 6–8 minutes, or until tender and lightly charred at the edges.

Mash together all the guacamole ingredients in a bowl until fairly well combined but still chunky. Season.

To serve, place the peppers, chicken and guacamole in a bowl, top with the soured cream, sprinkle with the grated cheese and paprika and serve, topped with coriander and wedges of lime.

Reduced-carb

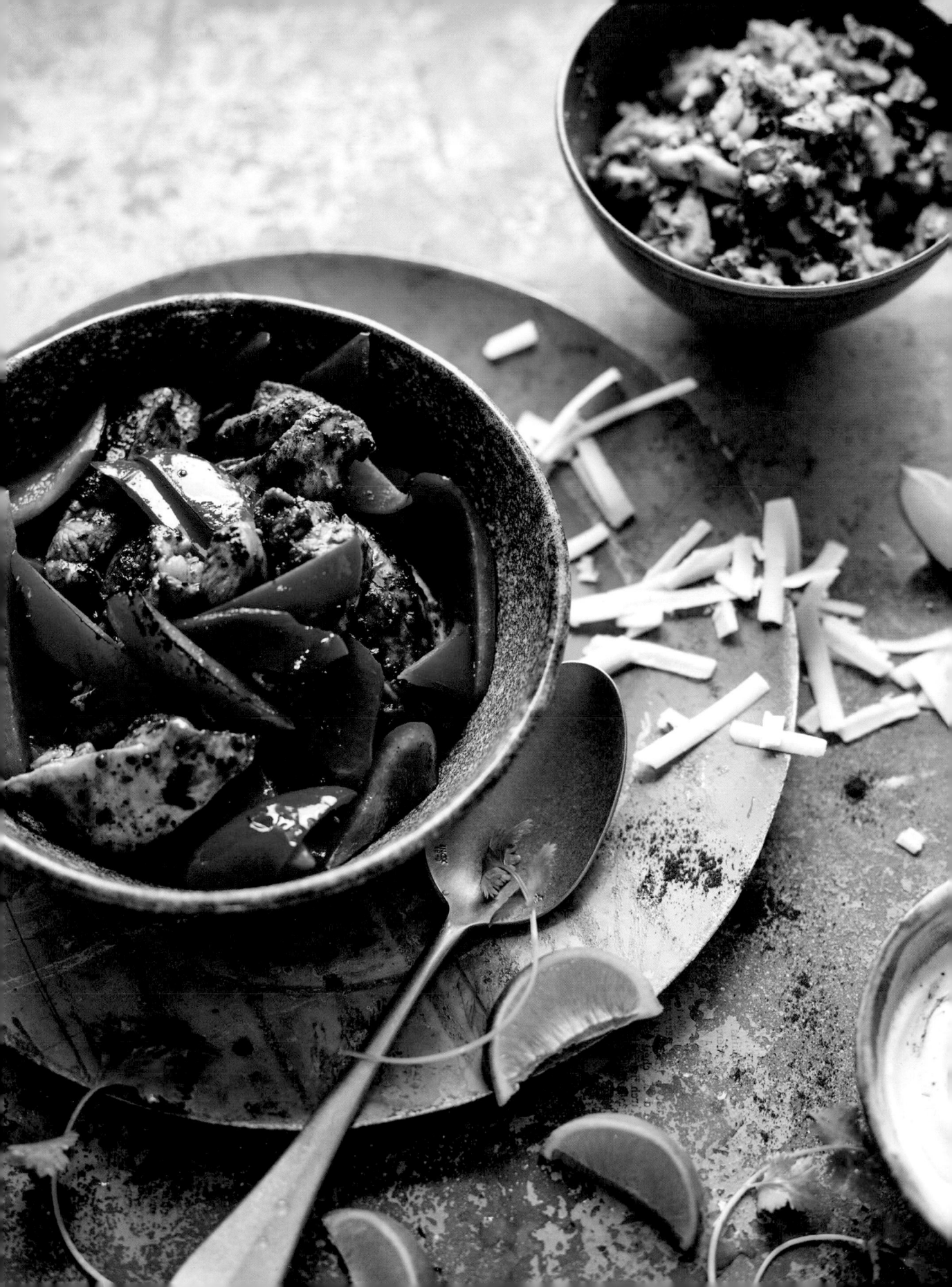

Ingredients

1 tbsp coconut oil
4 skinless chicken breast
   fillets, cut into 2cm dice
2 leeks, trimmed and
   thinly sliced
200g lean, thick-cut ham, cut
   into 1cm dice
1 x 300ml tub fresh
   chicken gravy
1 tbsp cornflour mixed with
   1 tbsp water
1 tbsp tarragon leaves, finely
   chopped
1 tbsp wholegrain mustard
100ml double cream
4 sheets of filo pastry
a little olive oil, for brushing
   (optional)
steamed greens, to serve

Tarragon Chicken, Ham and Leek Pie

Hold tight! Another pie for the win. In my first book it was Joe's chicken pie, then we had Joe's beef and mushroom pie, then Joe's fish pie in book 4. This is probably my favourite of them all. So tasty and perfect to enjoy with your friends or family.

Method

Preheat the oven to 200°C (fan 180°C/gas mark 6).

Melt the oil in a medium saucepan over a medium heat. Slide the chicken pieces into the pan. Fry gently for 2 minutes, then add the leeks and stir-fry for another 5 minutes until the chicken is cooked. Check by slicing into it to make sure the meat is white all the way through with no raw pink bits left.

Stir the ham and chicken gravy into the pan and bring to the boil. Stir in the cornflour mixture and chuck in the tarragon, mustard and cream. Bring the whole lot to the boil, then turn down the heat and simmer for 5 minutes, or until thickened.

Spoon the chicken filling into a medium ovenproof pie dish or four individual pie dishes. Cut the filo pastry into strips and scrunch them up slightly, then place them on top of the filling to cover it. Lightly brush the top of the pastry with olive oil, if using.

Bake in the oven for 10–12 minutes, until the sauce is bubbling and the filo pastry is crisp and golden brown. Serve with steamed greens of your choice.

Reduced-carb

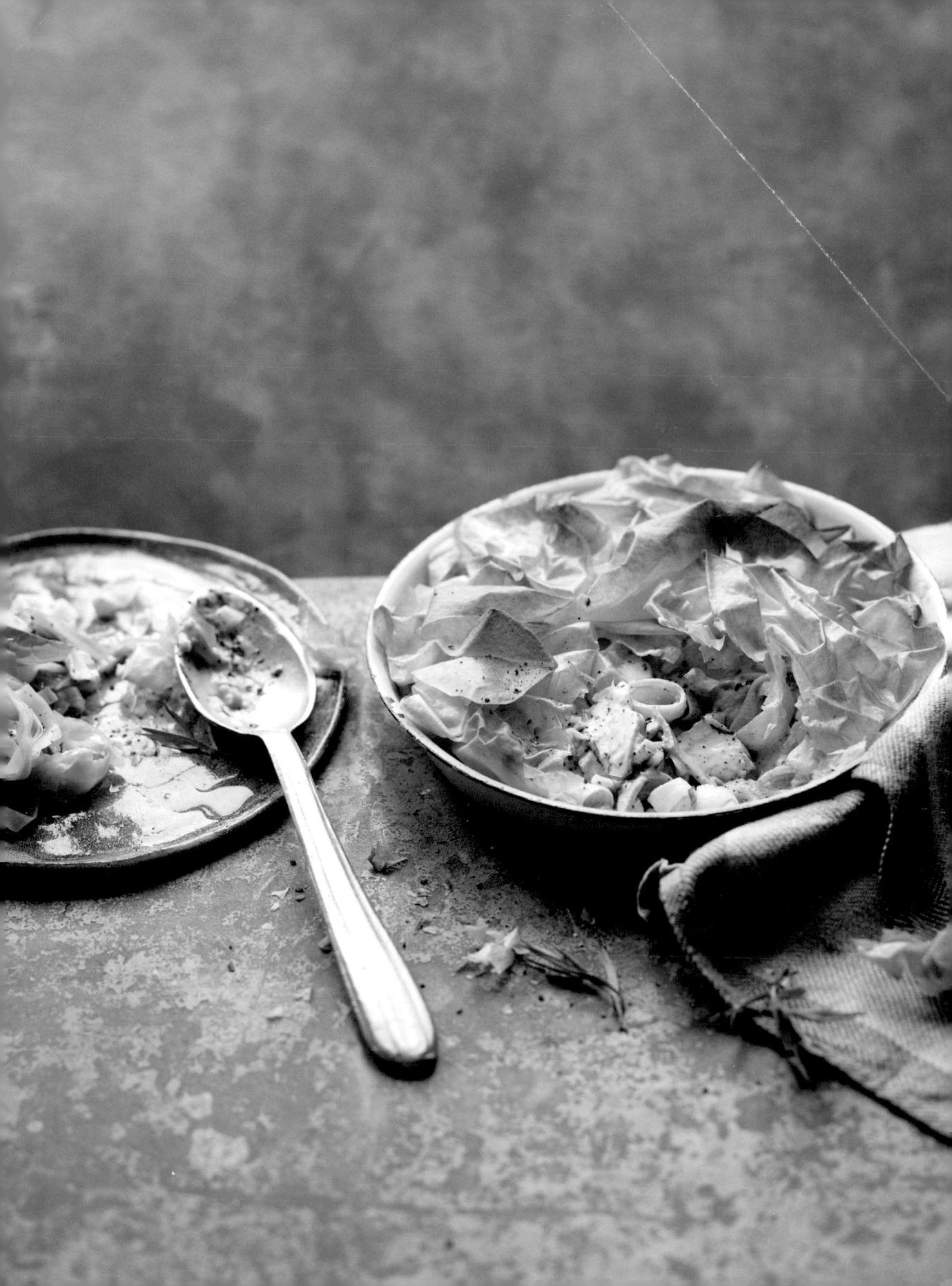

Longer recipe

Popcorn Chicken with Super Slaw

I love taking tasty fast-food ideas and making them into healthier Lean in 15 versions. This popcorn chicken tastes awesome and will satisfy your fried chicken craving.

Ingredients

4 tbsp cornflakes
3 tbsp tomato puree
1 tsp cayenne pepper
1 tsp garlic salt
2 tsp dried mixed herbs
black pepper
1 medium egg white
1 x 200g skinless chicken
  breast fillet

For the slaw

1 medium carrot, coarsely
  grated
100g green cabbage, finely
  shredded
½ red onion, thinly sliced
½ apple, cut into thin
  matchsticks
2 tbsp parsley, very finely
  chopped
¼ tsp toasted cumin seeds
2 tbsp apple cider vinegar

Method

Preheat the oven to 220°C (fan 200°C/gas mark 7).

Crush the cornflakes with a rolling pin until fine then transfer to a plate.

Mix the tomato puree, cayenne pepper, garlic salt and mixed herbs in a large bowl and season with pepper.

Whisk the egg white in a clean glass bowl until stiff peaks form, then fold it into the tomato puree mixture.

Cut the chicken into eight bite-sized pieces and dip the chicken into the egg mixture. Roll in the crushed cornflakes to coat evenly. Place the pieces in a shallow ovenproof dish in a single layer.

Bake in the oven for 15–20 minutes, or until lightly golden and crisp.

While the chicken is cooking, make the slaw by mixing together all the ingredients in a wide bowl. Season and serve with the popcorn chicken.

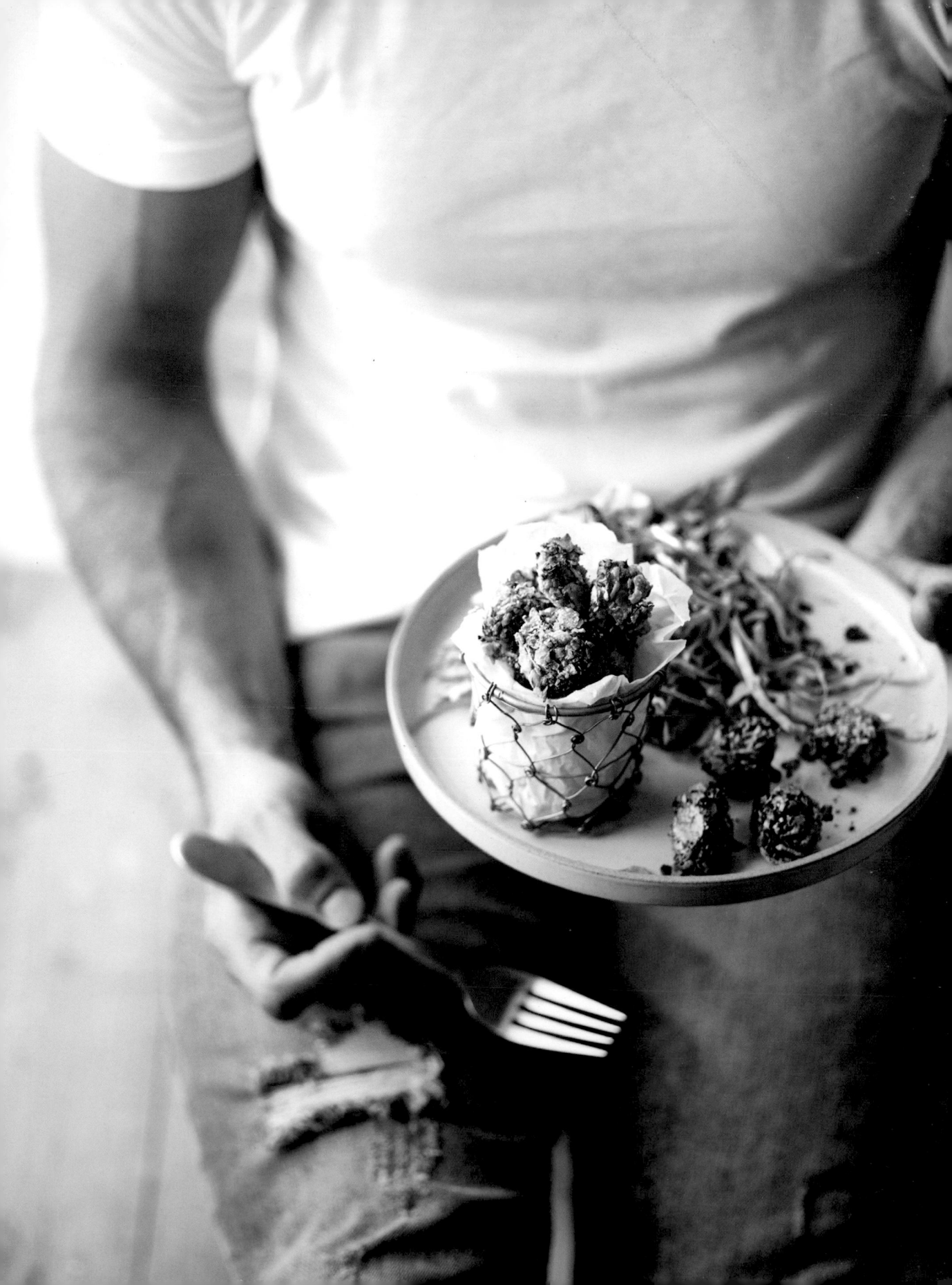

🕐 Make ahead

Ingredients

1 x 120g skinless salmon fillet,
  roughly chopped
100g raw peeled tiger prawns,
  roughly chopped
1 tbsp rose harissa spice paste
1 tbsp mint, finely chopped
2 tbsp coriander, finely
  chopped
zest of ½ lime
salt and pepper

For the salad

1 carrot, coarsely grated
¼ cucumber, peeled into
  thin shreds with a vegetable
  peeler
½ small red onion, finely
  chopped
1 tbsp each of mint
  and coriander, chopped, plus
  extra leaves to serve
2 tsp rose harissa paste
juice of ½ orange
1 clove garlic, crushed
1 tbsp each of toasted pumpkin
  and sunflower seeds (optional)
1 tbsp toasted pine nuts

Moroccan Salmon and Prawn Fish Cakes

These are the best fish cakes I've ever made. Serve with a super-tasty seed and nut salad, which is full of healthy fats to fuel your body.

Method

Preheat the grill to medium-high.

Place the salmon, prawns, harissa, mint, coriander and lime zest in a food processor. Season and pulse until well combined, but still a little chunky.

Divide the mixture into three portions and form each one into a patty, about 1.5cm thick.

Place on a grill rack and cook under the grill for about 6–8 minutes, turning halfway through, or until cooked and lightly golden.

Meanwhile, make the salad by chucking the carrot, cucumber, red onion and chopped herbs into a bowl. Whisk together the harissa with the orange juice and garlic and pour over the vegetables. Season well and toss to combine.

Pile on a plate with the seeds (if using) and pine nuts and serve with the fish cakes.

Reduced-carb

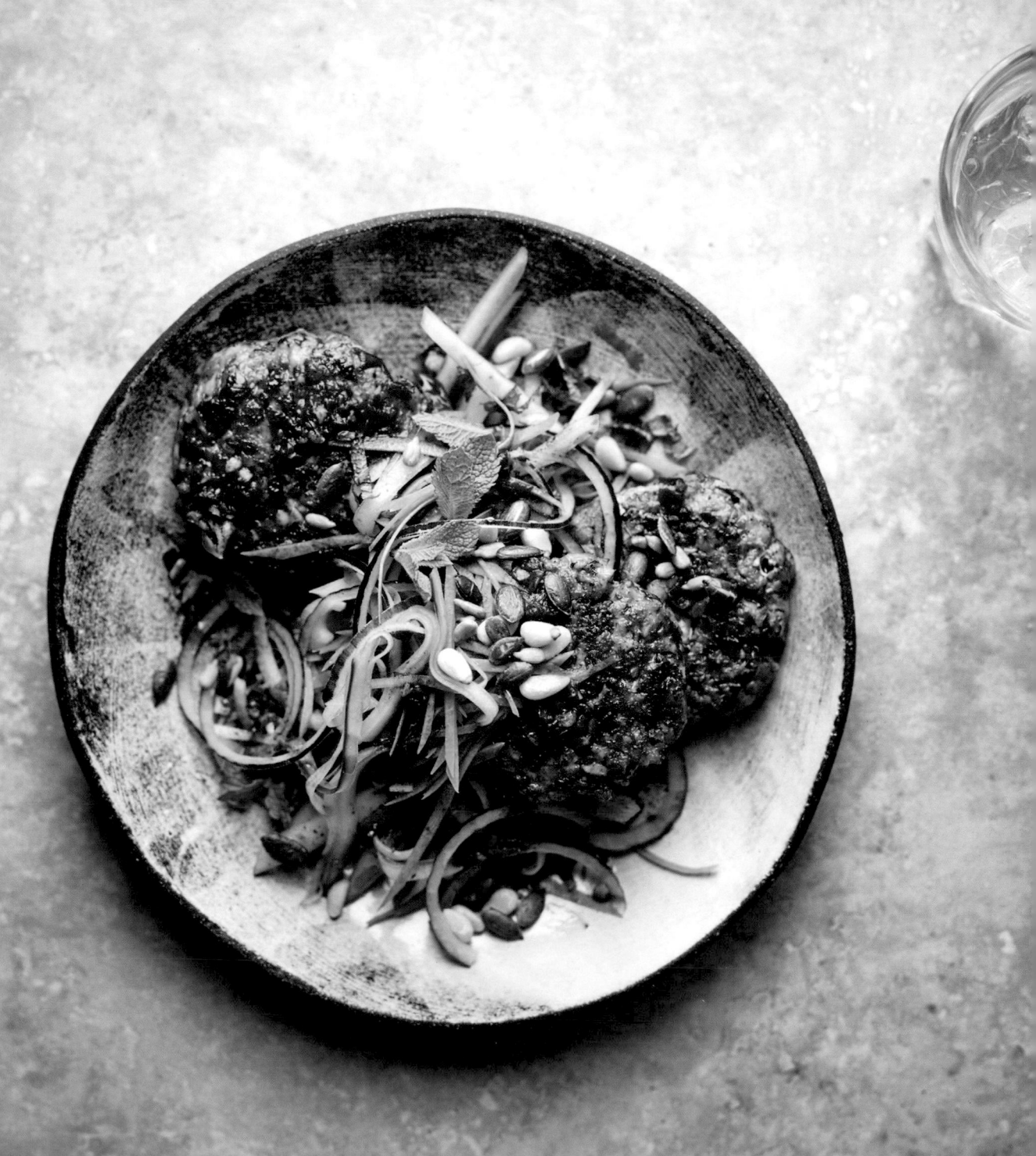

Green Chicken Masala Curry with Kachumber Salad

Next time you fancy ordering a take-away curry, give this one a go instead. It tastes authentically Indian and will keep you on track to getting lean. Kachumber is a mix of finely chopped fresh vegetables served as a side.

Ingredients

4 tbsp coriander (leaves and stalks), finely chopped
2 tbsp mint leaves, chopped
1 tsp finely grated ginger
1 tsp finely grated garlic
1 small onion, finely chopped
1 tbsp mild curry powder
200ml chicken stock
200ml coconut milk
½ tbsp coconut oil
250g skinless, boneless chicken thighs, cut into bite-sized pieces
1 courgette, cut into 1.5cm dice
salt and pepper

For the kachumber salad

¼ cucumber, finely diced
1 ripe plum tomato, finely diced
¼ red onion, finely diced
½ green chilli, de-seeded and finely diced
2 tbsp coriander, chopped, plus extra for garnish
juice of 1 lime, plus extra wedges to serve

Method

Place the chopped herbs, ginger, garlic, onion, curry powder, stock and coconut milk in a small food processor and blend until fairly smooth.

Melt the oil in a large non-stick frying pan. Add the chicken and courgette and stir-fry for 2–3 minutes.

Pour over the herb mixture, bring to the boil and simmer for 10–12 minutes, or until the chicken is cooked through and tender. Season well.

Meanwhile, mix all the ingredients for the kachumber salad in a bowl, season and serve with the chicken curry. Top with coriander sprigs and serve with wedges of lime.

Reduced-carb

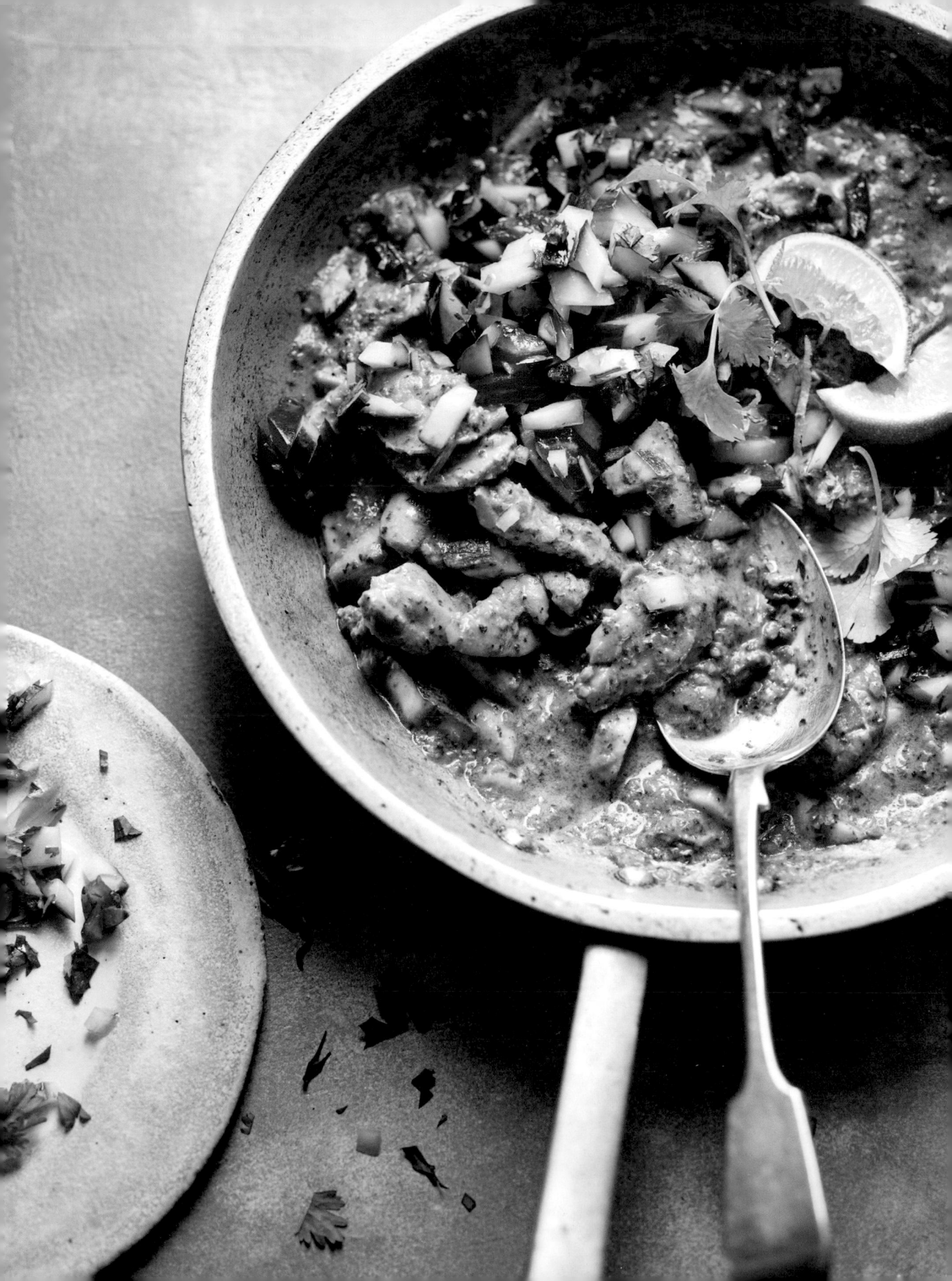

Tandoori Chicken Shish Kebabs with Minty Raita Dip

This will make a great Friday night feast when you're craving a kebab. Chicken mince is easy to find now, but if you can't buy it, you could also use turkey mince.

Ingredients

225g lean chicken mince
1 tbsp tandoori spice mix
juice of ½ lemon, plus extra
   slices to serve
1 tbsp natural or Greek-
   style yoghurt
1 tsp finely grated ginger
1 clove garlic, crushed
1 tbsp coriander, finely
   chopped, plus extra
   for garnish
big green salad, to serve
pinch of chilli powder, to serve

For the raita

¼ cucumber, de-seeded and
   finely diced
1 tomato, finely diced
2 tbsp mint leaves, finely
   chopped
juice of 1 lime
6 tbsp natural or
   Greek-style yoghurt
pinch of ground cumin
salt and pepper

Method

Make the raita by stirring all the ingredients in a bowl until well combined. Season and chill until ready to serve.

Slide the chicken mince, tandoori spice mix, lemon juice, yoghurt, ginger, garlic and coriander into a bowl, season and mash it together using your fingers until well combined.

Divide the mixture into three portions and press each portion onto a metal skewer to form a sausage shape.

Preheat the grill to medium.

Place the skewers under the grill and cook for 8–10 minutes, turning halfway through, until lightly browned and cooked all the way through.

Serve the shish kebabs with the raita and a big green salad. Sprinkle over the chilli powder and top with the chopped coriander. Serve with lemon slices.

Reduced-carb

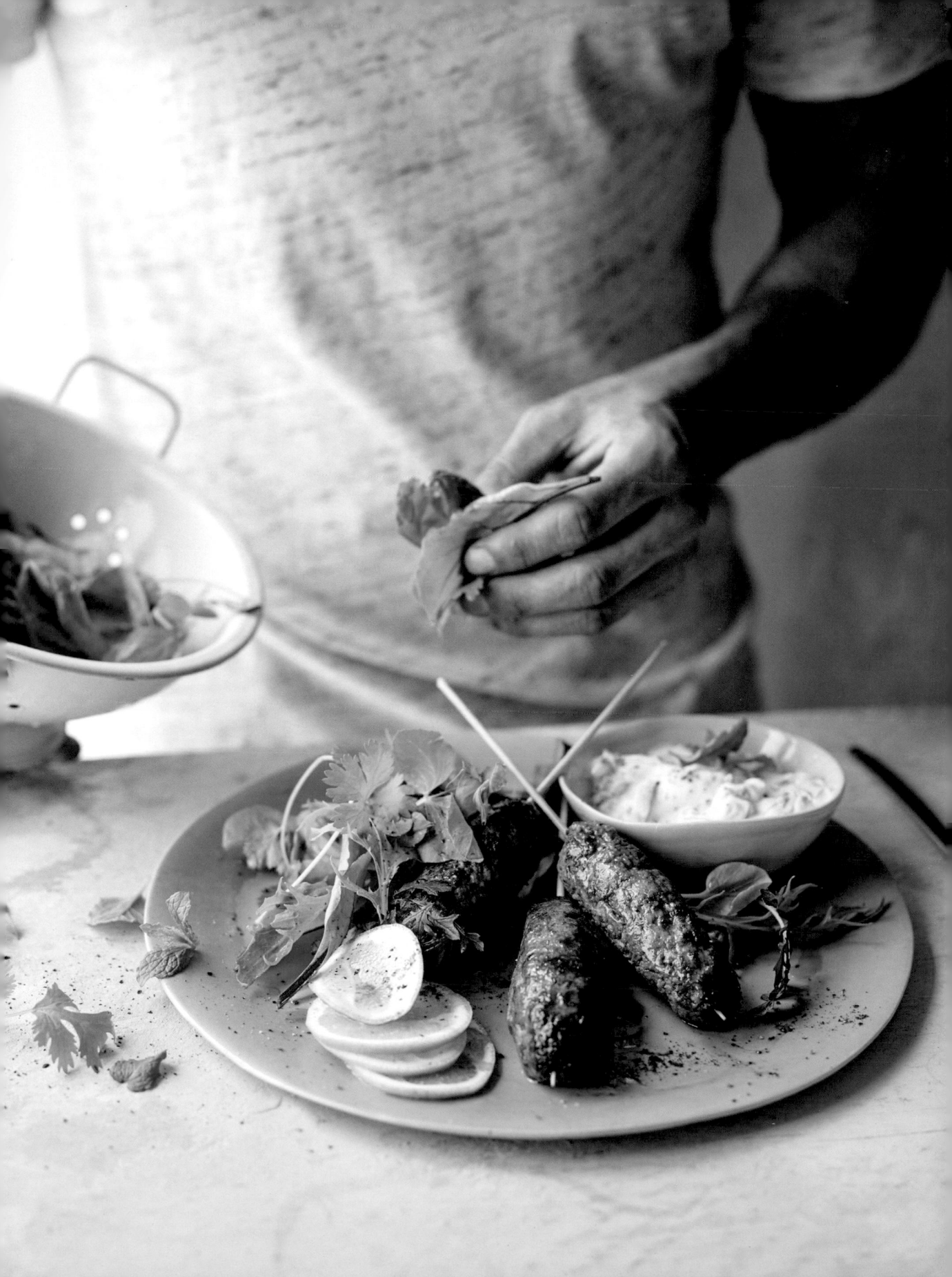

Lamb Kofte Tagine

This is a recipe that once you try it, you'll be making it again very soon. It's got so much flavour and is really simple to make.

Ingredients

1 tbsp coconut oil

250g shop-bought lamb meatballs

½ onion, grated

2 cloves garlic, grated

1 tsp grated ginger

1 tsp ground cumin

¼ tsp ground cinnamon

1 tsp sweet smoked paprika

250g passata

2 tbsp tomato puree

1 tbsp preserved lemon, chopped

75ml chicken or vegetable stock

salt and pepper

100g chickpeas

5–6 black pitted olives

2 tbsp natural yoghurt, whisked

small bunch of chopped coriander leaves

Method

Melt the oil in a wide non-stick frying pan over a high heat.

Add the meatballs and brown for 2–3 minutes on all sides.

Stir in the onion, garlic, ginger, spices, passata, puree, preserved lemon and stock. Season and bring to a rapid boil. Cook, stirring occasionally for 8–10 minutes or until thickened and the meatballs are cooked through.

Stir in the chickpeas and olives and cook for 3–4 minutes more.

Remove from the heat, dollop with the yoghurt, scatter with the coriander and enjoy.

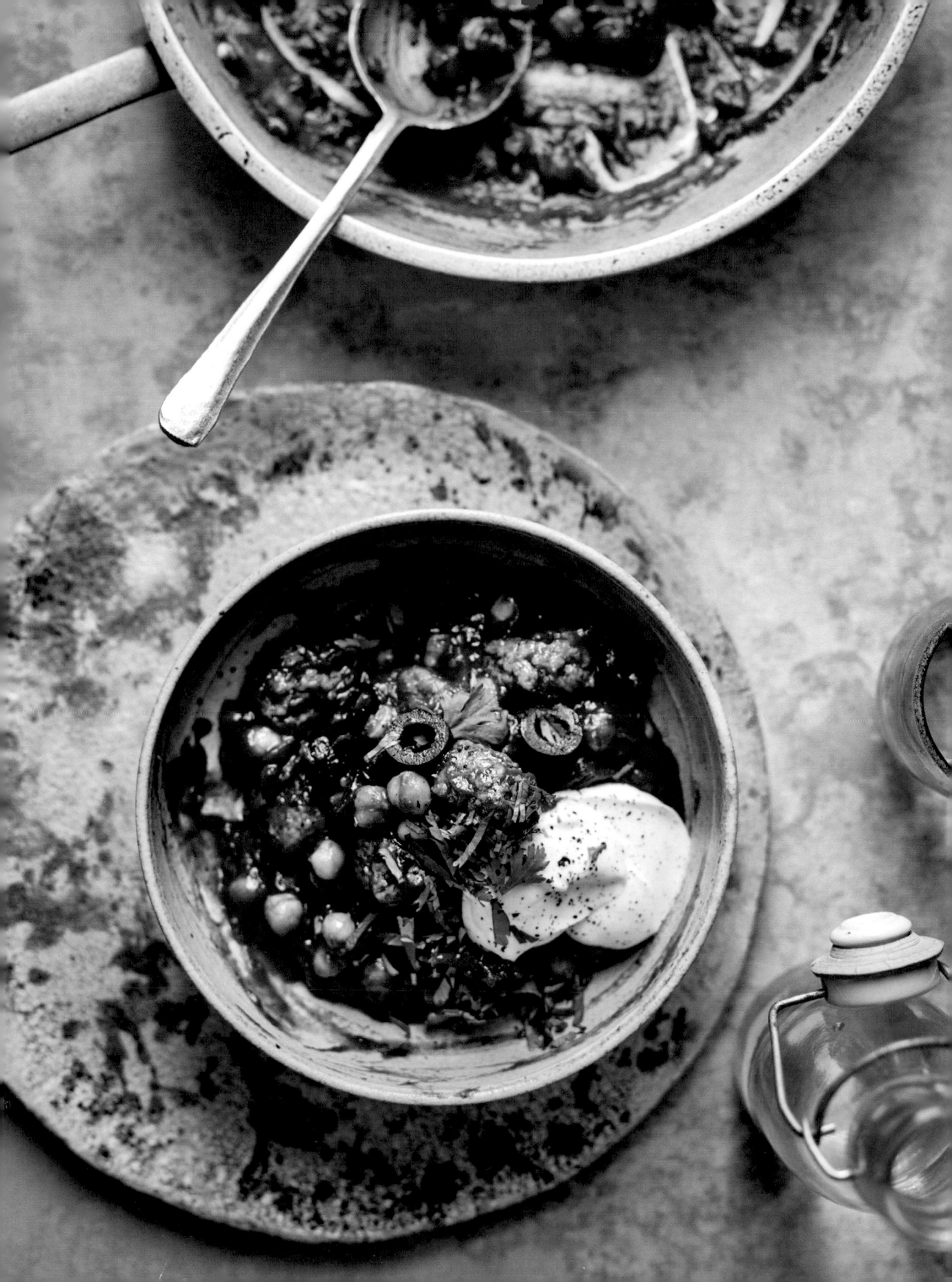

5
Post
Workout
Recipes

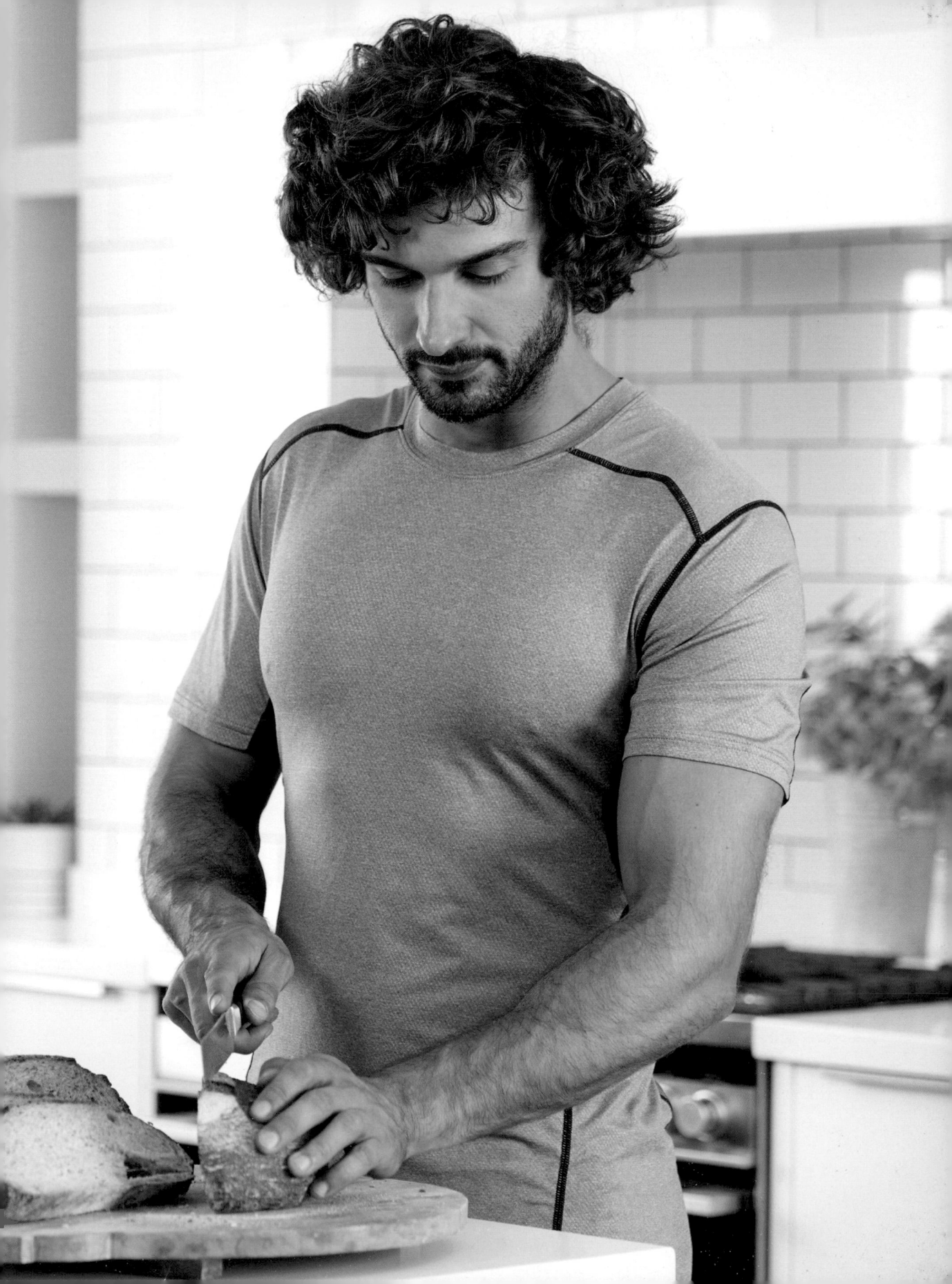

Coconut and Berry Compote Porridge

There's nothing better than a big bowl of warm oats after a workout. This recipe is so satisfying and will refuel your body.

Ingredients

¼ tsp cardamom
  seeds, crushed
500ml almond milk
a few drops of vanilla
  extract
80g quinoa
50g porridge oats
150g mixed berries
  (raspberries, blackberries,
  blueberries), plus a few extra
  to serve
2 tbsp mixed seeds
  (flaxseeds, pumpkin
  seeds, sunflower seeds),
  to serve (optional)
2 tbsp coconut flakes, to serve

Method

Place the cardamom seeds and almond milk in a saucepan with the vanilla extract and quinoa. Bring to the boil, then lower the heat. Simmer, lid-off, for 15 minutes, or until the quinoa tails sprout.

Add the oats and 80ml water to the pan and cook for about 10 minutes, uncovered, until thick and porridge-like. Add more water if it becomes too thick.

Meanwhile, make a quick berry compote by adding the berries to a pan with 1 tablespoon of water. Simmer for 4–5 minutes, covered. Mix well and mash with a fork until the berries have broken down.

Mix half the compote with the porridge and divide between two bowls. Drizzle over the rest of the compote. Top with the mixed seeds (if using), more fresh mixed berries and coconut flakes, and serve.

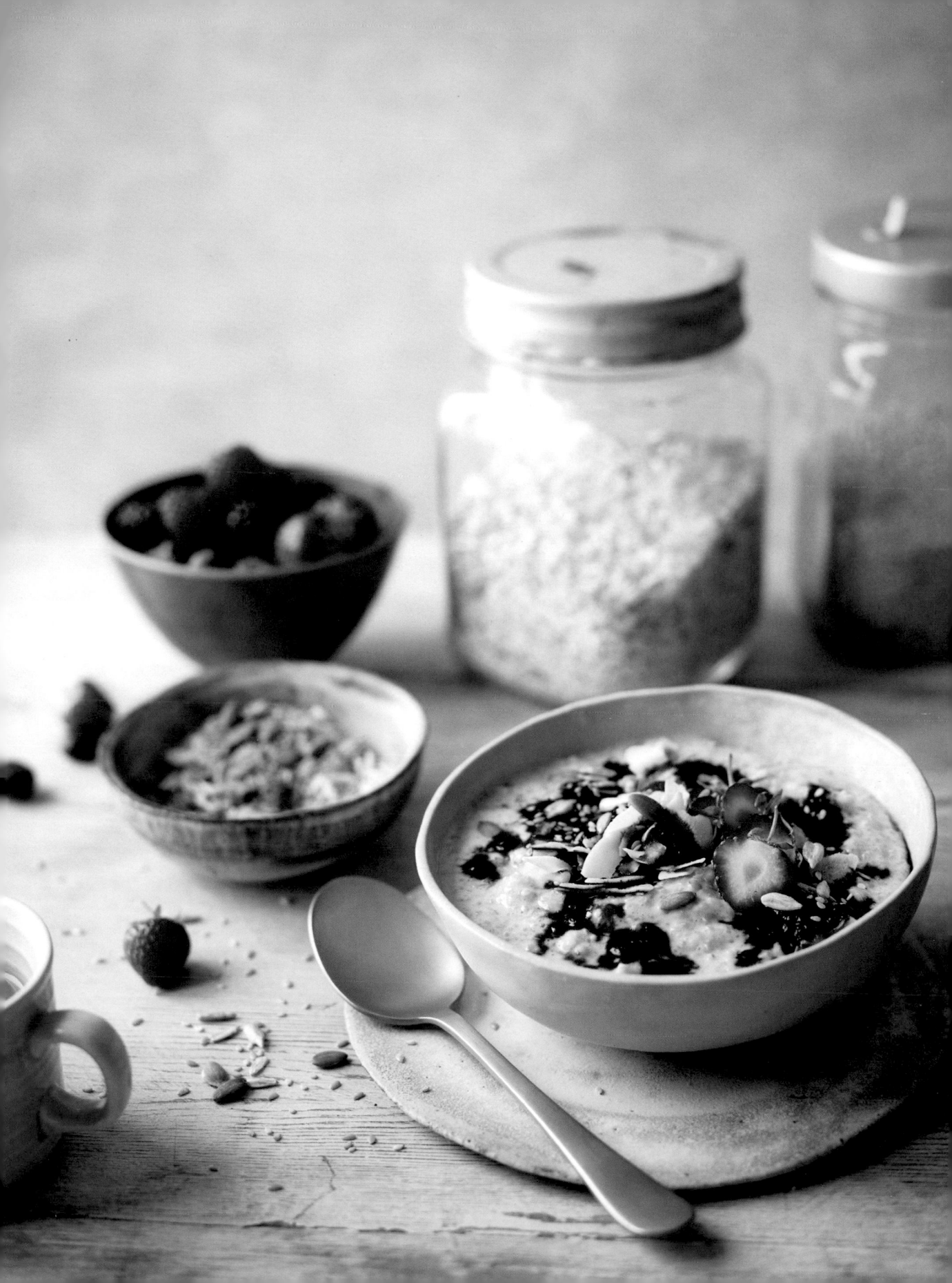

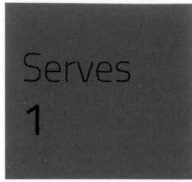

Joe's Bounty Overnight Oats

For those who follow me on social media you'll know I'm pretty much obsessed with these overnight oats. They taste like a Bounty chocolate bar so it feels like a treat. You can make them the night before and store in the fridge for up to 2 days.

Ingredients

1 banana, roughly broken
250ml almond milk
100ml coconut milk
1 scoop (30g) chocolate protein powder
1 tbsp cocoa powder
100g rolled oats

To serve

1 tsp chia seeds (optional)
2 tsp desiccated coconut
handful of blackberries

Method

Blend the banana, almond and coconut milk, protein powder and cocoa into a blender. Blend until smooth.

Pour into a container and stir through the oats, making sure they are well coated. Cover with a lid and place in the fridge for 8 hours or overnight.

In the morning, transfer the oats into a bowl, loosening them with 2 tablespoons of water if the texture is thicker than you would like it.

Decorate with chia seeds (if using), desiccated coconut and blackberries and serve immediately.

Post-workout

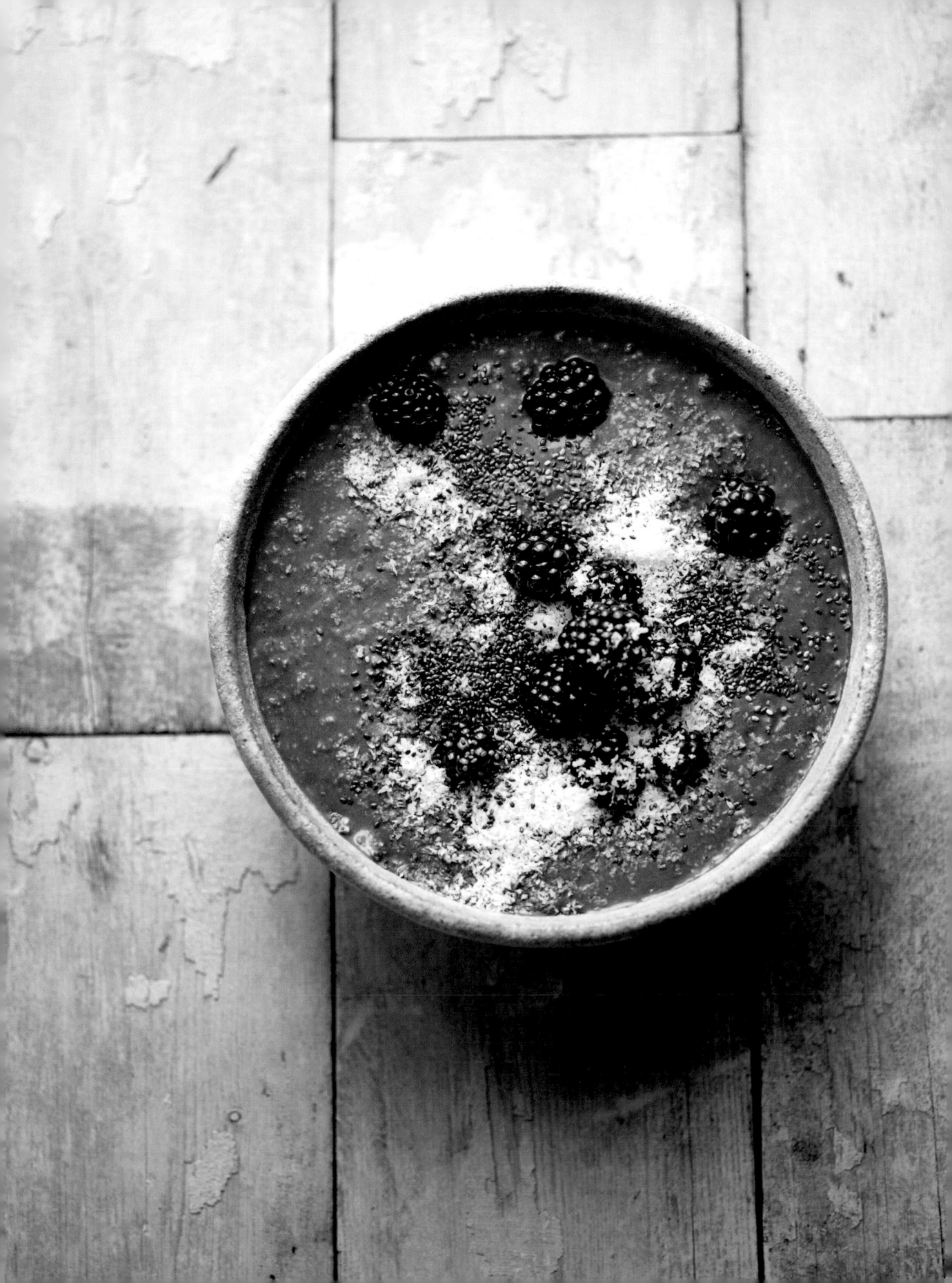

Raspberry, Banana and Buttermilk Pancakes

This recipe is great if you have a sweet tooth at breakfast. As you can see, the camera always eats first, so be sure to post your pancake pics with the hashtag #Leanin15.

Ingredients

120g self-raising flour
pinch of ground cinnamon
1 tbsp golden caster sugar
1 tsp baking powder
1 tbsp protein powder
1 large egg
100ml buttermilk, plus extra
  (optional)
100g raspberries
½ banana, roughly chopped
1 tbsp coconut oil, melted
runny honey, for drizzling
  (optional)

Method

Place the self-raising flour in a mixing bowl with the cinnamon, golden caster sugar, baking powder and protein powder. Stir to mix well.

In a bowl, whisk the egg and gradually stir in the buttermilk. Add to the dry ingredients, whisking to combine evenly to make a smooth batter (add a little extra buttermilk if the batter is too thick).

In a bowl, mix the raspberries and chopped banana together.

Pour the batter into a measuring jug. Brush some of the coconut oil on the base of a non-stick frying pan (about 12–14cm in size) and place over a medium to high heat.

Pour one-third of the batter into the pan and cook for 3–4 minutes. Scatter one-third of the raspberry and banana mixture over the top.

Flip the pancake over and cook for 1–2 minutes, or until lightly golden and cooked through.

Repeat with the remaining batter and raspberry and banana mixture to make three pancakes in total. Serve the pancakes stacked, with a drizzle of honey, if desired.

Post-workout

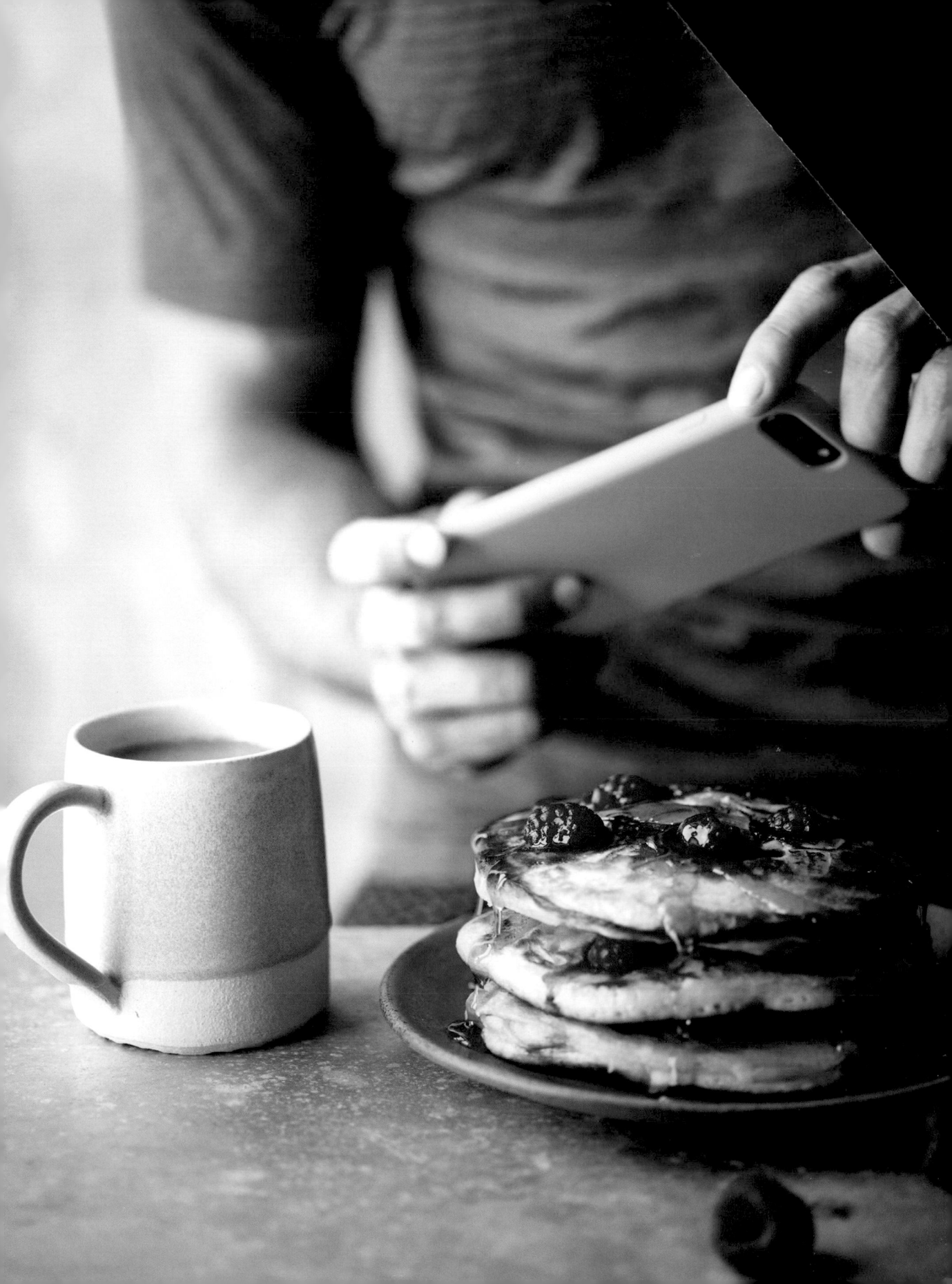

Coconut and Lime Pancakes

Another pancake recipe? Guilty. I can't deny it, I love pancakes. These ones will put a big smile on your face.

Ingredients

125g white spelt flour
2 tsp baking powder
25g dessicated coconut, plus
  extra for garnish (optional)
pinch of salt
2 medium eggs, beaten
100ml almond milk
1 tsp vanilla extract
1 tsp finely grated lime zest,
  plus extra for garnish
  (optional)
2 tbsp coconut oil
maple syrup, for drizzling
  (optional)

Method

Place the flour, baking powder and coconut in a wide mixing bowl with the pinch of salt.

In a large measuring jug, whisk together the eggs, almond milk, vanilla and lime zest and slowly pour into the flour mixture and whisk until combined. If you have time, let the batter rest in the fridge for about 30 minutes.

When you're ready to cook, heat a little of the oil in a large non-stick frying pan.

Pour three ladlefuls of the batter (about 3 tablespoons each) into the pan, well spaced apart. Cook the pancakes over a medium heat for 2–3 minutes and then flip over and cook for 2 minutes on the other side.

Repeat with the remaining batter, placing the cooked pancakes in a low oven while you cook the rest.

Serve the pancakes drizzled with a little maple syrup and top with extra lime zest and coconut, if desired.

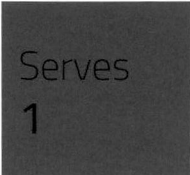

Serves
1

Joe's Post-workout Shake

This is something I usually have just after my workout as a supplement. This doesn't count as a meal, though, so I recommend making another meal from this section about an hour after your session.

Ingredients

1 scoop (30g) chocolate
  protein powder
large handful of spinach
4 ice cubes
1 tsp runny honey
1 ripe banana, broken
  into pieces
300ml water

Method

Place all ingredients into a blender and blend until smooth.

Enjoy right away, or drink when chilled.

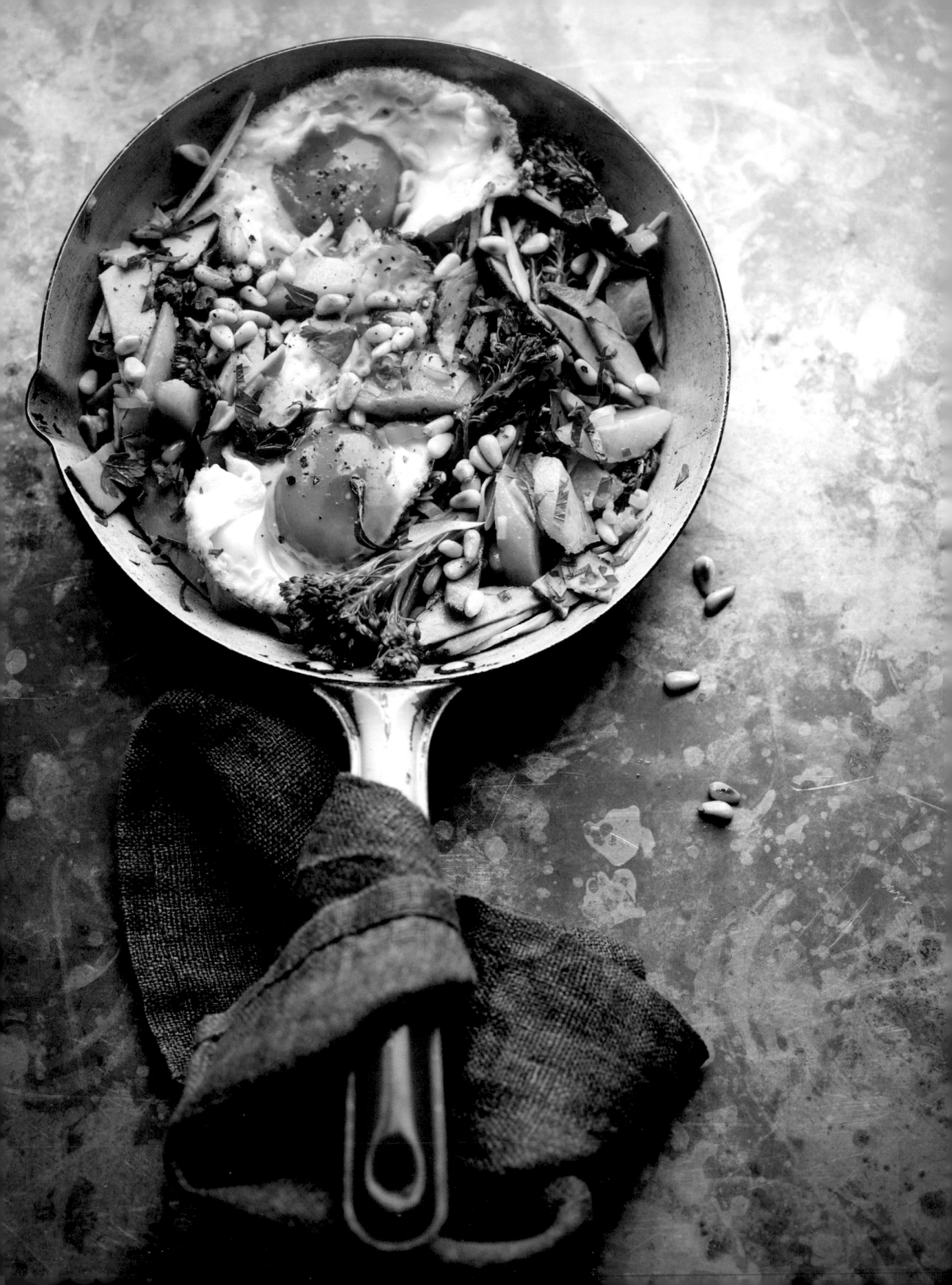

Joe's Mcleanie Breakfast Hash

Oooh this breakfast is a bit of me. Forget about unhealthy cereal or croissants on the move, this is quick, easy and will get you lean.

Ingredients

30g midget trees (tenderstem broccoli), thinly sliced
½ tbsp coconut oil
1 large potato, peeled, cooked and roughly chopped (about 200g)
1 clove garlic, crushed
4 spring onions, finely sliced
¼ courgette, coarsely grated
large handful of baby spinach leaves, chopped
salt and pepper
3–4 thick slices of lean deli-style ham, roughly chopped (about 180g)
2 tbsp parsley, finely chopped
2 medium eggs
1 tbsp toasted pine nuts, to scatter (optional)

Method

Simmer the broccoli in a small sauccpan of boiling water for 2 minutes. Drain and roughly chop.

Melt the oil in a wide non-stick frying pan and add the potato, garlic, spring onions and courgette. Stir and cook for 5–6 minutes over a high heat.

Stir in the spinach and cook for a further 2 minutes, or until just wilted.

Season the mixture and stir in the chopped ham, broccoli and parsley.

Make two dips in the hash and crack an egg into each one. Put a lid on the pan and cook until the egg is just set or cooked to your liking. Season and serve scattered with the toasted pine nuts, if using.

Smoked Salmon and Poached Egg Benedict

This makes a perfect weekend brunch. I love inviting friends over and making this one for them.

Ingredients

large handful of baby
  spinach leaves
1 medium egg
¼ tsp coconut oil
3 spring onions, sliced
salt and pepper
1 tbsp light mayonnaise
1 tsp Dijon mustard
1 tsp hot vegetable or
  chicken stock
1 thick slice of toasted rye
  bread (or sourdough or
  good white)
100g sliced smoked salmon
1–2 tsp dill or chives,
  finely chopped, to serve

Method

Simmer the spinach in a saucepan of boiling water for 1–2 minutes, or until just wilted. Drain in a sieve, pressing down with the back of a spoon, and discard excess liquid. Roughly chop and set aside.

Meanwhile, poach the egg by bringing a pan of water to the boil. Crack in the egg and poach at a gentle simmer for 3–4 minutes, or until cooked to your liking.

Melt the oil in a non-stick frying pan and add the spring onions and the drained spinach. Season, stir and cook for 2–3 minutes until warmed through.

In a small bowl, whisk together the mayonnaise, mustard and the stock until smooth.

Chuck the toast on a plate and top with the spinach and the smoked salmon.

Top with the poached egg and drizzle over the mustard sauce. Sprinkle over the dill or chives, then season to taste and tuck in.

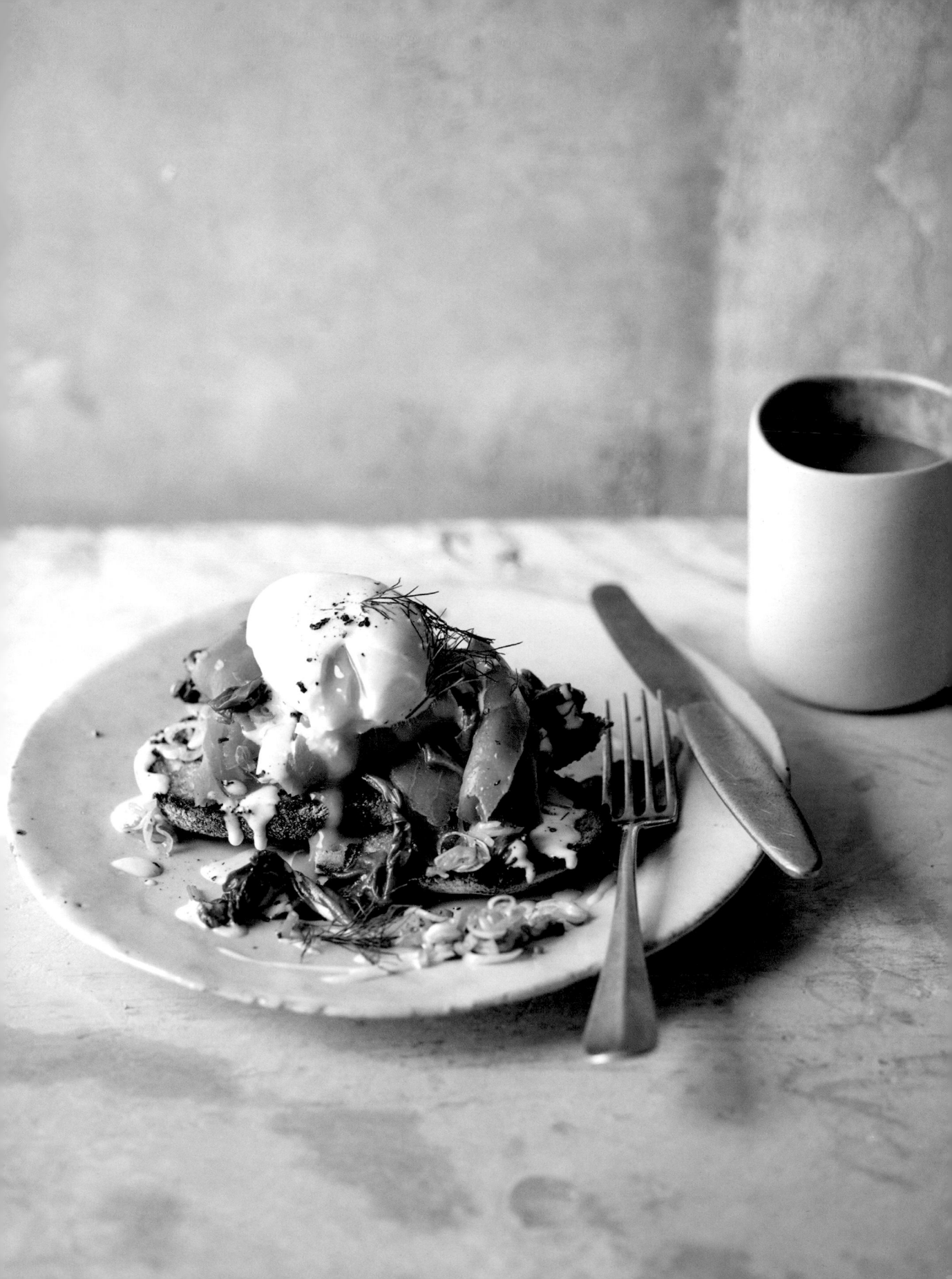

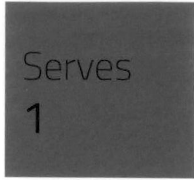
Herbed Omelette, Ham and Rocket Wraps

This is an awesome breakfast or lunch idea. It tastes good hot or cold so you can always wrap it in foil and take it to work for lunch.

Ingredients

2 large eggs
salt and pepper
½ tbsp coconut oil
2 tbsp chopped mixed herbs of your choice (chives, parsley, tarragon, basil, dill)
2–3 slices thick deli-style ham, roughly chopped
1 large flour tortilla wrap
small handful of wild rocket
1 plum tomato, finely chopped

Method

Place the eggs in a bowl and whisk lightly to combine. Season well.

Melt the oil in medium non-stick frying pan over a medium to high heat. Add the egg mixture and, as the base begins to set, sprinkle the herbs and ham on top, and continue to cook until the top is set. Remove from the heat and keep warm.

Heat the tortilla wrap in a hot griddle pan or large frying pan for a minute on each side, or warm it in a microwave for a few seconds until warm.

To serve, place the warmed wrap on a board and slide the omelette on top. Lay the rocket and tomato down the centre, then roll up and eat.

Post-workout

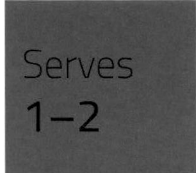

Serves
1–2

Make ahead

Roasted Pepper, Bacon, Kale and Potato Frittata

This is another recipe that you can eat hot or cold like a Spanish omelette. I often make two at a time and store one in the fridge for lunch the following day, served with a side salad.

Ingredients

4 large eggs
2 tbsp milk
salt and pepper
½ tbsp coconut oil
½ small onion, very finely diced
200g cooked, peeled potatoes, cut into 1.5cm pieces
1 clove garlic, crushed
1 red chilli, finely diced – remove the seeds if you don't like it hot
4 rashers of lean bacon (all visible fat removed), chopped
2 jarred red peppers, drained and roughly chopped
30g kale, finely shredded

Method

Preheat the grill to medium-high.

In a medium bowl, whisk the eggs and milk together. Season and set aside.

Melt the oil in a non-stick frying pan over a medium heat. Add the onion, potatoes, garlic red chilli, bacon, red peppers, chilli and chopped bacon. Sauté for 3 minutes, until the onion is translucent. Add the kale and cook until it wilts, about 5 minutes.

Reduce the heat slightly and add the eggs to the pan mixture. Cook for about 4 minutes until the bottom and edges of the frittata start to set.

Slide the frittata under the grill and cook for 6–8 minutes until the top is set and golden. Slice and serve.

Breakfast Ham and Chicken Club 'Sub'

This recipe is the cover star of this book and for good reason. Just look at it. How can you not want to eat that after a workout? It's the dream.

Ingredients

½ x 200g skinless chicken breast fillet
½ tbsp coconut oil, plus extra for frying
3 tbsp tomato puree
1½ tbsp fat-free Greek-style yoghurt
2 tbsp sweet chilli sauce
few drops each of Worcestershire and Tabasco sauce
2 rashers of lean bacon (all visible fat removed)
1 medium egg
1 large sub roll
2–3 little gem lettuce leaves, roughly torn
½ cucumber, finely sliced
3 tomatoes, finely sliced

Method

Place the chicken between two pieces of cling film, and using a rolling pin or wooden mallet, lightly beat until slightly thinned to an even thickness.

Melt the coconut oil on a hot griddle pan and cook the chicken for 6–8 minutes on each side, until cooked through. Check by slicing into it to make sure the meat is white all the way through, with no raw pink bits left. Set aside.

Preheat the grill to medium-hot. Meanwhile, in a small bowl, mix together the tomato puree, yoghurt and sweet chilli sauce. Stir through the Worcestershire sauce and Tabasco sauce.

Grill the bacon until crispy and set aside.

Melt 1 tsp of the coconut oil in a non-stick frying pan and fry the egg until cooked to your liking. Set aside.

Halve the sub roll and lightly toast both of the cut sides.

Place the base of the sub roll on a board, toasted side up. Spread with half the tomato puree mixture, then top with the lettuce, cucumber and tomato slices.

Shred the chicken and chuck on with the grilled bacon and finally the fried egg.

Spread the remaining tomato puree mixture over the toasted side of the top piece of the roll, sandwich together and get stuck in.

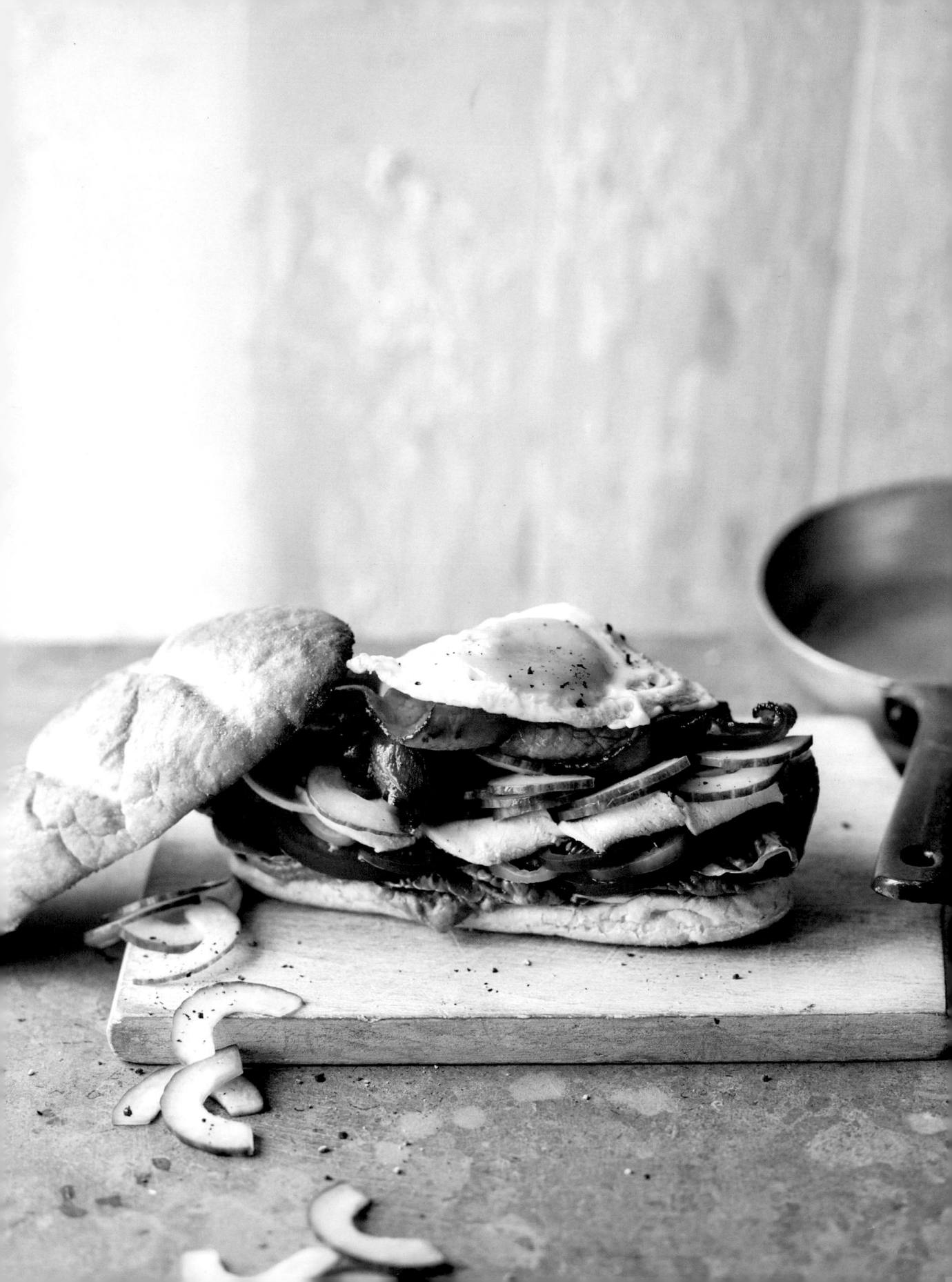

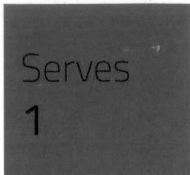

Korean Minced Chicken and Noodle Stir-fry

I love the flavours in this recipe. Your local butcher can easily mince chicken breast for you but if not, simply chop a breast into squares and blitz it in a food processor yourself.

Ingredients

200g fresh egg noodles
10g fresh beansprouts
½ tbsp coconut oil
250g chicken or turkey mince
4 spring onions, sliced into
  3cm diagonal lengths
2 cloves garlic, crushed
100g midget trees (tenderstem
  broccoli), thinly sliced
½ red pepper, de-seeded and
  thinly sliced
½ yellow pepper, de-seeded
  and thinly sliced
1 tbsp dark soy sauce
2 tsp Korean red pepper paste
  (Gochujang) or hot chilli sauce
1 tbsp sweet chilli sauce

Method

Place the noodles and beansprouts in a heatproof bowl. Cover with boiling water. Stand for 2–3 minutes or until tender. Separate the noodles using a fork, and drain.

Meanwhile, heat a non-stick frying pan or wok over a high heat. Melt half of the oil, swirling to coat the pan. Stir in the chicken mince.

Cook, stirring with a wooden spoon to break up the mince, for 4–5 minutes or until browned and just cooked through. Transfer the mince to a bowl.

Add the remaining oil to the pan, and swirl to coat. Add the spring onions and garlic and stir-fry for 30 seconds, thenadd the broccoli and peppers and stir-fry for 3–4 minutes until tender.

Return the mince to the pan with the soy sauce, Korean pepper paste and sweet chilli sauce, and stir-fry for 1 minute. Add the cooked noodles and beansprouts, stir to combine, then transfer to a bowl and dig in.

Post-workout

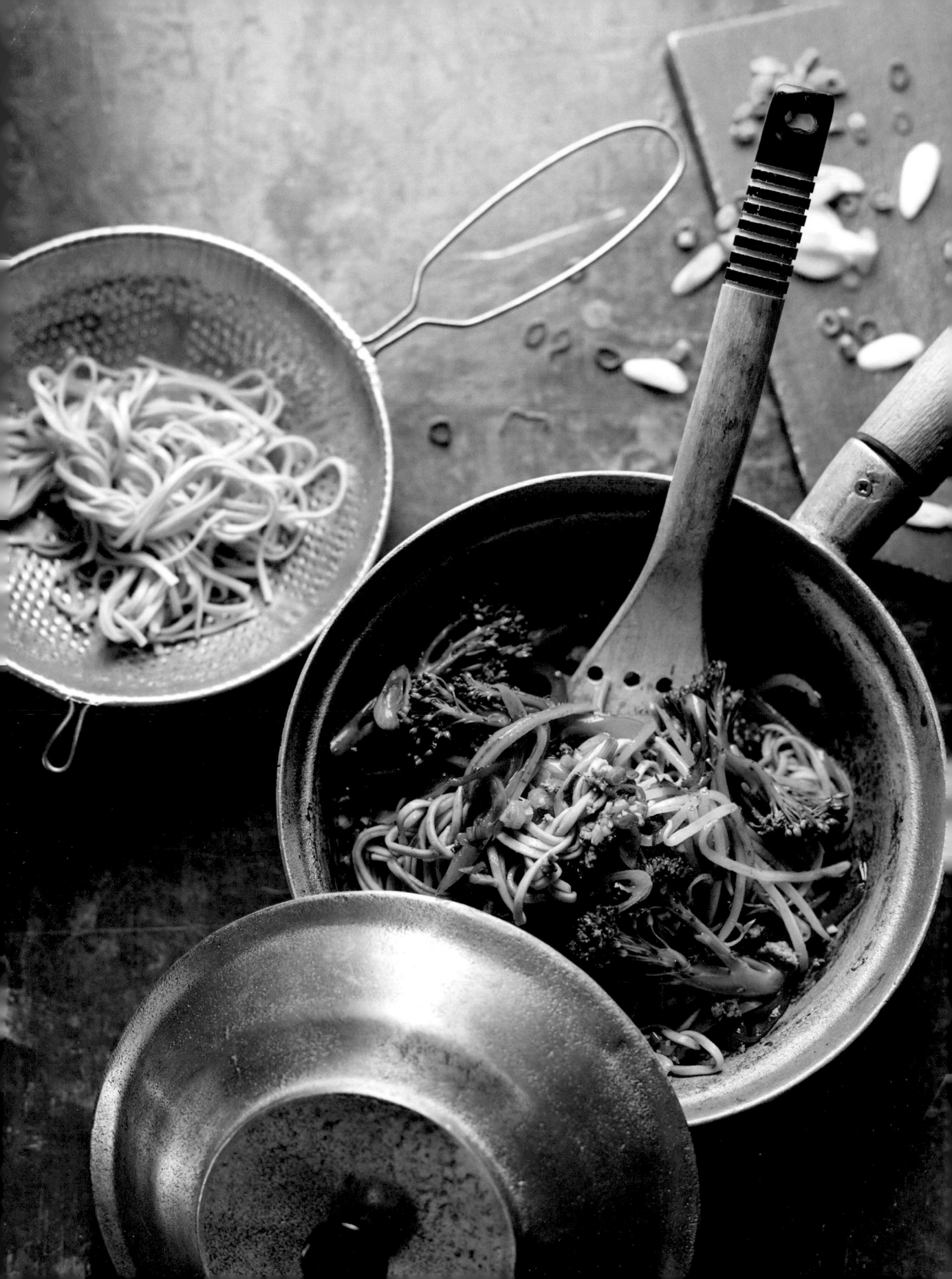

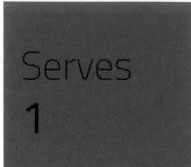

Prawn, Chilli and Tomato Linguini

Lots of people think pasta should be cut out completely when trying to lose weight. Your muscles actually need to be replenished with carbohydrates after you exercise, so don't fear pasta. If you enjoy eating it, go for it.

Ingredients

100g fresh or dried linguini
½ tbsp coconut oil
1 shallot, finely chopped
2 cloves garlic, crushed
1 red chilli, finely diced
200g raw peeled tiger prawns
8 cherry tomatoes, chopped
small handful of wild rocket,
  roughly chopped
1 tsp lemon juice, plus lemon
  wedges to serve

Method

Cook the linguini according to packet instructions and drain.

Melt the oil in a non-stick frying pan and fry the shallot and garlic for 1–2 minutes, or until softened.

Add the chilli and prawns, and cook, stirring constantly, until the raw grey colour of the prawns turns pink, which shows you they are cooked.

Add the tomatoes and cook for 2–3 minutes, then stir in the rocket and lemon juice. Add the cooked linguine and toss to coat evenly. Pile the linguine onto a plate and serve with lemon wedges.

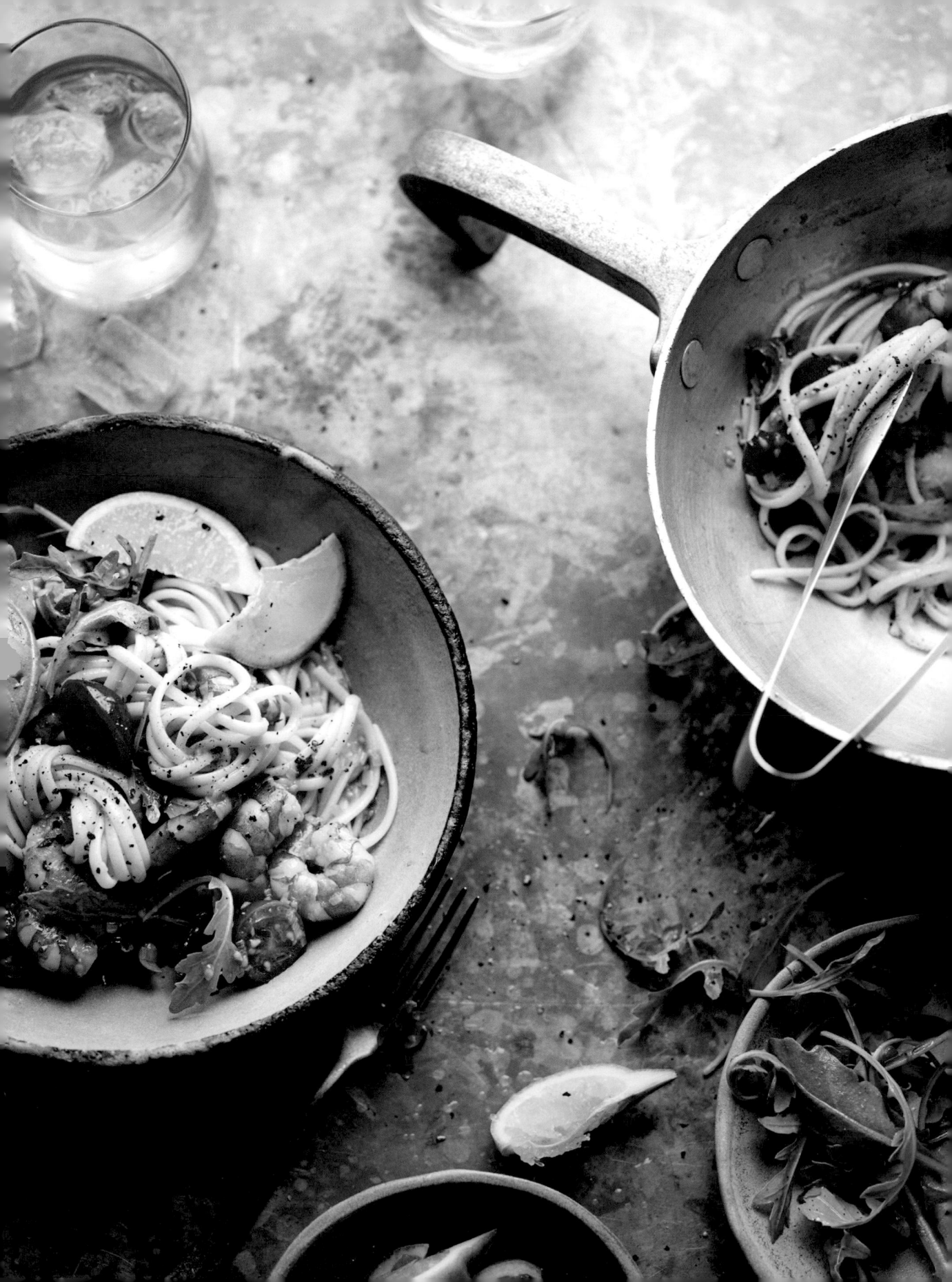

Speedy On-the-Hob Chicken Lasagne

This is such a simple way of making a lasagne and getting all those lovely flavours but without waiting hours for it to bake in the oven. Give it a go. You'll be surprised at how simple it is and how great it tastes.

Ingredients

1 tbsp coconut oil

3–4 chicken sausages (about 250g), skinned and roughly crumbled

2 shallots, finely chopped

100g fresh lasagne sheets, cut into large bite-sized squares

½ x 400g tin of chopped tomatoes

200g onion-and-garlic flavoured passata

1 tsp golden caster sugar

¼ tsp dried red chilli flakes

salt and pepper

1–2 tbsp oregano or parsley, chopped

Method

Melt the oil in a medium non-stick frying pan over a high heat and add the chicken sausage meat and shallots. Stir-fry for a few minutes until the meat is sealed.

Stir in the lasagne pieces, chopped tomatoes, passata, sugar, chilli flakes and 100ml water. Season well, cover and bring to the boil.

Allow to cook for 10–12 minutes, until the pasta is cooked through and the sauce has thickened.

Remove from the heat, scatter over the chopped herbs and serve immediately, straight from the pan.

Post-workout

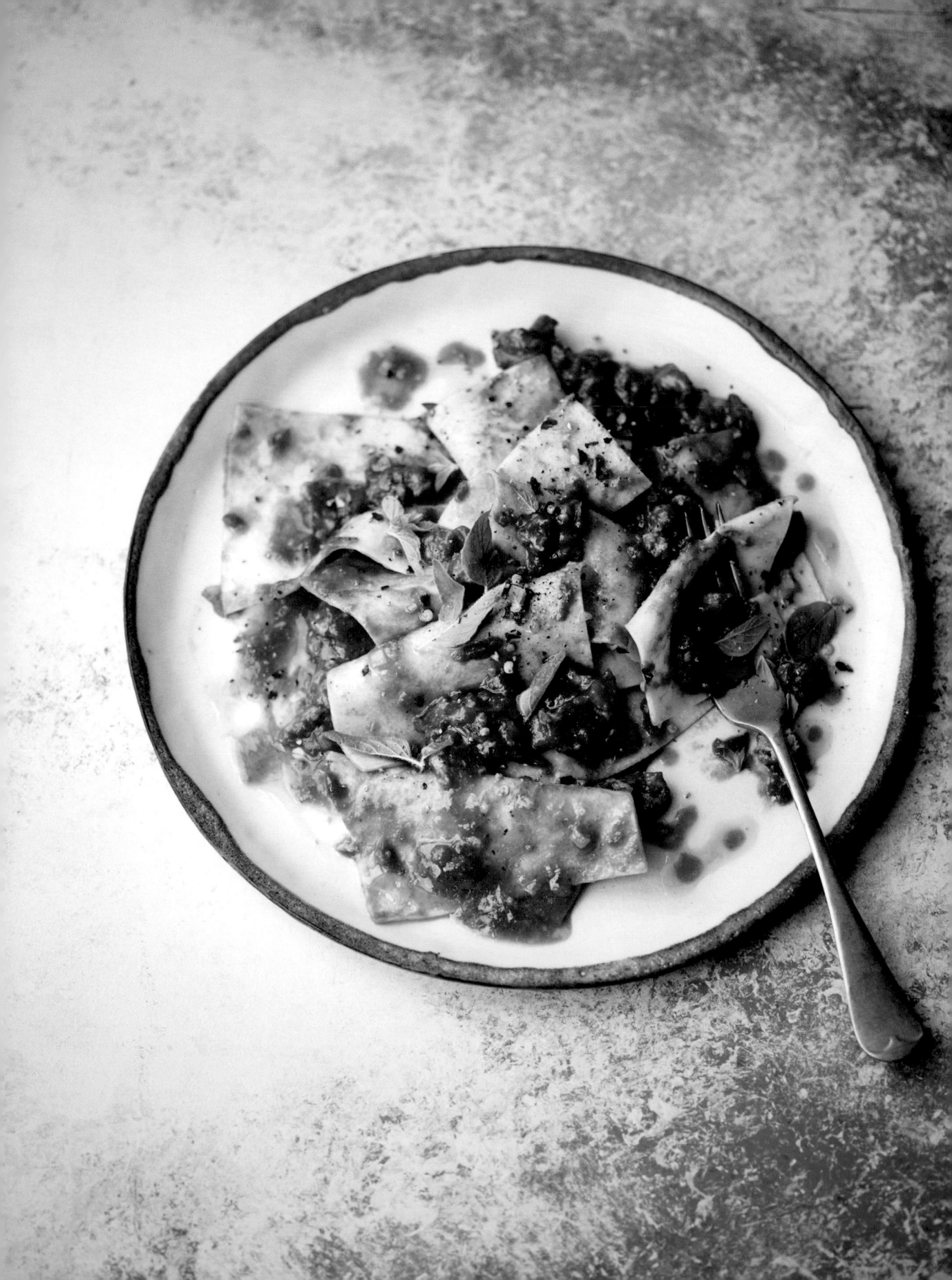

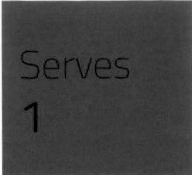

Japanese Prawn and Soba Noodle Salad

This makes a nice change from a traditional salad. The dressing tastes incredible with the prawns.

Ingredients

100g dried soba noodles
½ cucumber, de-seeded and finely diced
4 spring onions, thinly sliced on the diagonal
250g cooked, peeled tiger or jumbo prawns
4 tbsp coriander leaves, finely chopped
1 tsp toasted sesame seeds

For the dressing

1 tbsp mirin
2 tbsp apple cider vinegar
1 tbsp light soy sauce
1 tsp very finely grated ginger
1 tsp runny honey
few drops of sesame oil
black pepper

Method

Cook the soba noodles in a large saucepan of boiling water until just tender (2–4 minutes) or according to packet instructions. Drain and refresh under cold running water.

For the dressing, whisk the ingredients in a bowl until smooth. Season with the pepper and pour the dressing over the cooked soba noodles.

Chuck in the cucumber and spring onions and toss to combine, then serve topped with the prawns, coriander and sesame seeds.

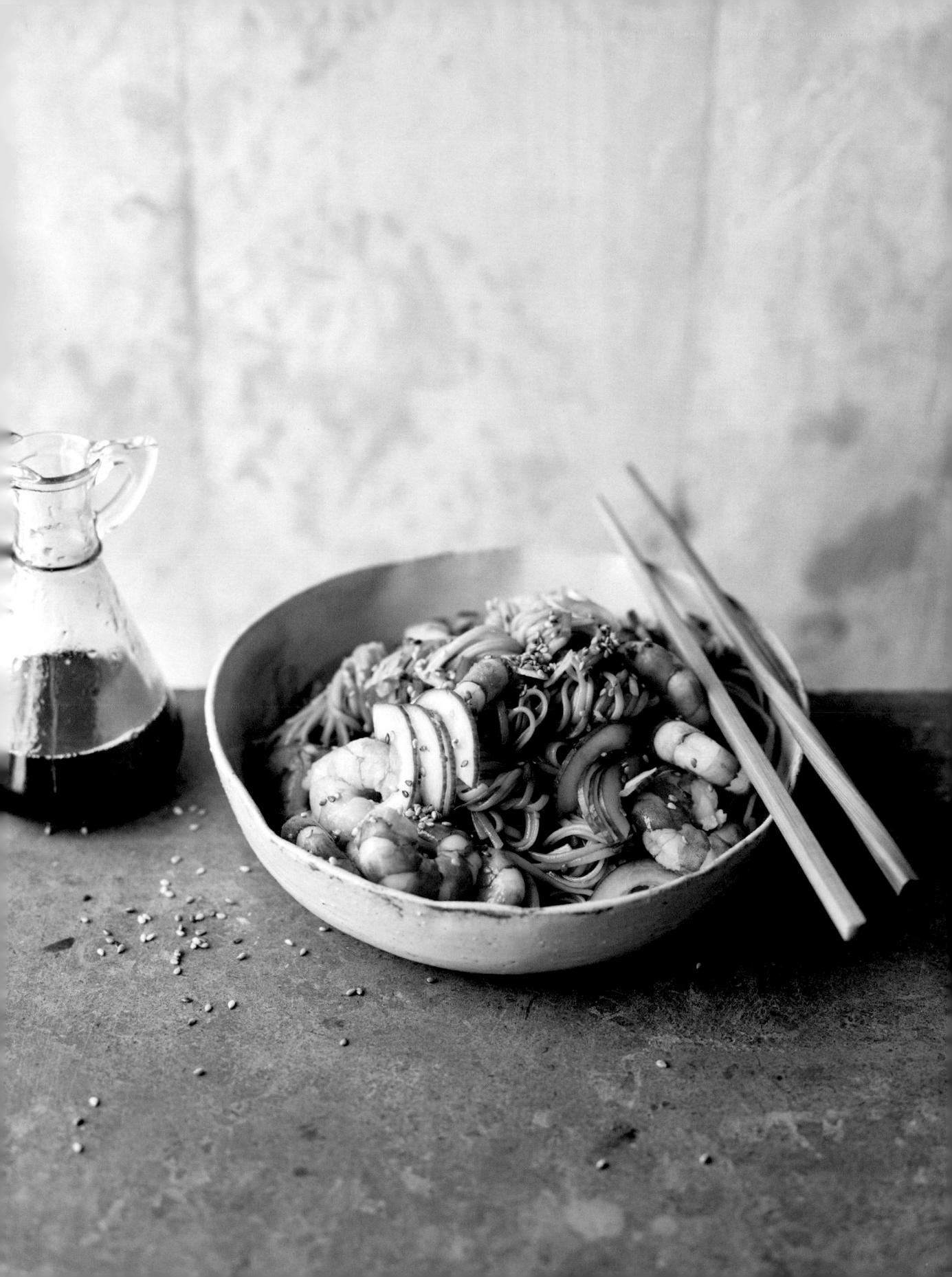

Pork Bibimbap Bowl

Bibimbap is a Korean word that means 'mixed rice'. This version uses pork but you could use chicken breast instead.

Ingredients

½ tbsp coconut oil
180g lean pork tenderloin, very thinly sliced
1 small carrot, peeled
¼ courgette
4 shiitake mushrooms
6 sugarsnap peas
salt
1 medium egg (optional)
small handful of baby spinach leaves
175g pre-cooked brown basmati rice
roughly chopped spring onion and red chilli, for garnish (optional)

For the sauce

1 tsp Korean hot pepper paste (gochujang) or hot chilli sauce
1 tbsp apple cider vinegar
1 tsp runny honey
¼ tsp each of finely grated garlic and ginger
1 tbsp dark soy sauce

Method

Melt half of the coconut oil in a large non-stick frying pan over a high heat.

Add the pork in a single layer and cook for 1–2 minutes on each side, or until cooked through. Set aside.

Slice the carrot and courgette into thin matchsticks, and the mushrooms and sugarsnaps into thin slices.

Heat a clean large non-stick frying pan with a lid and add the remaining oil. Stir-fry the mushrooms for 4 minutes then push to the side of the pan as far away from the heat as possible. Fry the carrots for 2 minutes, then push into a pile next to the mushrooms. Add the courgette to the pan and fry for 2 minutes, then push to the side of the pan next to the carrots.

Add piles of the sugarsnaps and spinach to the pan, then cover with the lid, remove from the heat and allow to sit for 2–3 minutes, until the spinach is wilted.

If you are serving with a poached egg, poach the egg in a saucepan of gently simmering water for 4 minutes, or until cooked to your liking. Drain.

Mix all the ingredients for the sauce and set aside.

Place the cooked brown rice in the middle of the bowl, and place the vegetables and pork on top in separate piles.

Drizzle the bibimbap sauce over the top and serve. Mix thoroughly before topping with the chopped spring onion, red chilli and the poached egg, if using.

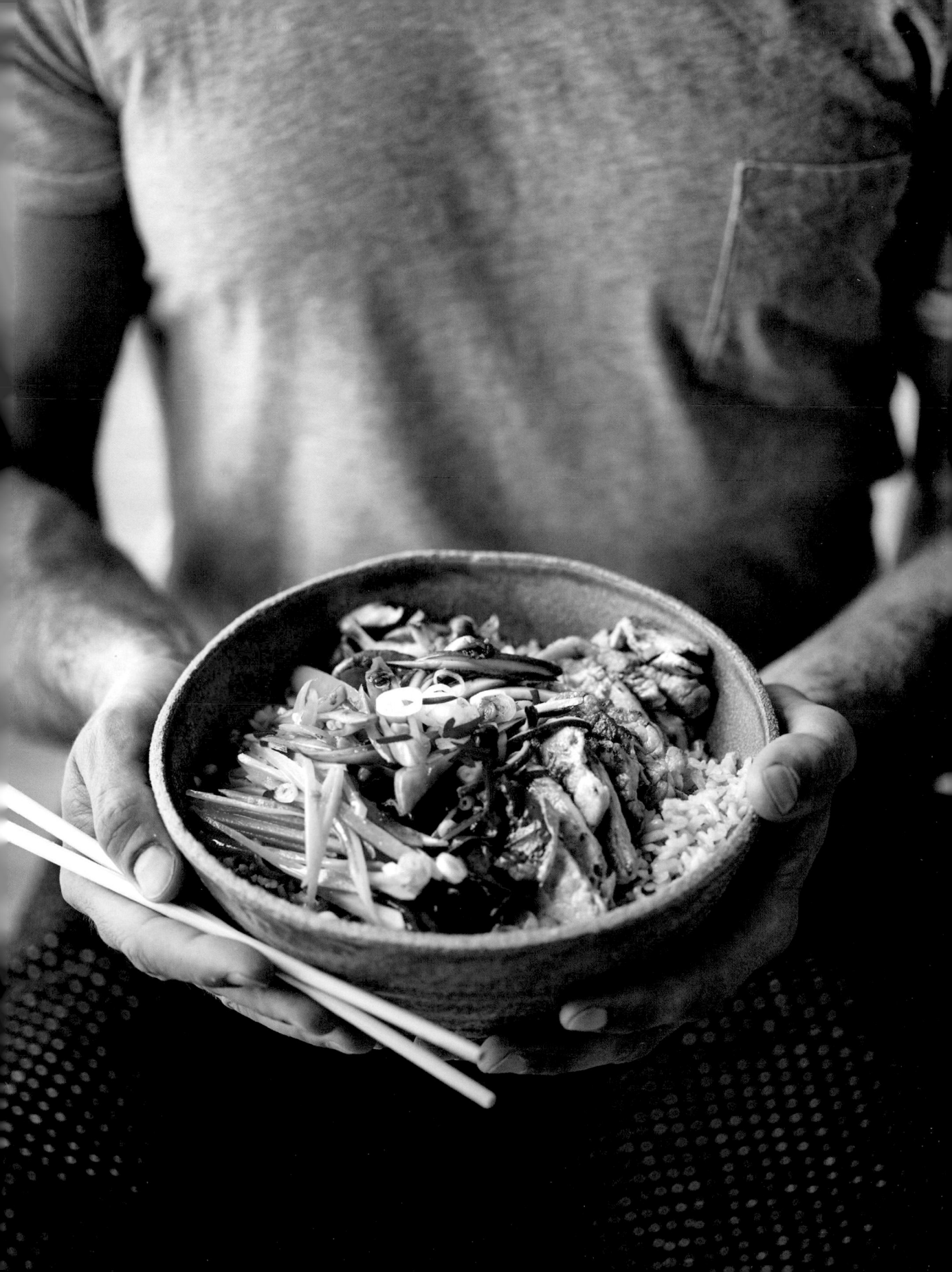

Chicken, Pea and Kale Orzo

If you've not tried orzo pasta before you really should give this recipe a go. This is a bowl of goodness that I'm sure you'll love and will make more than once.

Ingredients

1 x 200g skinless chicken
  breast fillet
1 tbsp coconut oil
4 spring onions, sliced
salt and pepper
600ml boiling hot vegetable
  or chicken stock
100g dried orzo pasta
100g frozen peas
40g kale, shredded
finely grated zest and juice
of 1 lemon, plus sliced
  zest for garnish (optional)
small handful of mint,
  chopped

Method

Place the chicken between two pieces of cling film, and using a rolling pin or wooden mallet, lightly beat until slightly thinned to an even thickness.

Melt ½ tablespoon of the coconut oil on a hot griddle pan and cook the chicken for 6–8 minutes on each side, until cooked through. Check by slicing into it to make sure the meat is white all the way through, with no raw pink bits left. Set aside.

Melt the remaining coconut oil in a large non-stick saucepan. Add three-quarters of the sliced spring onions with a pinch of salt and stir-fry for 1–2 minutes.

Add the boiling hot stock and the orzo. Cover and boil for 8 minutes, then chuck in the peas and kale, season, and simmer for another 4 minutes, until the pasta is cooked and the kale has wilted.

Shred the cooked chicken and add to the orzo with the lemon zest, juice and mint. Top with the remaining spring onion and extra lemon zest.

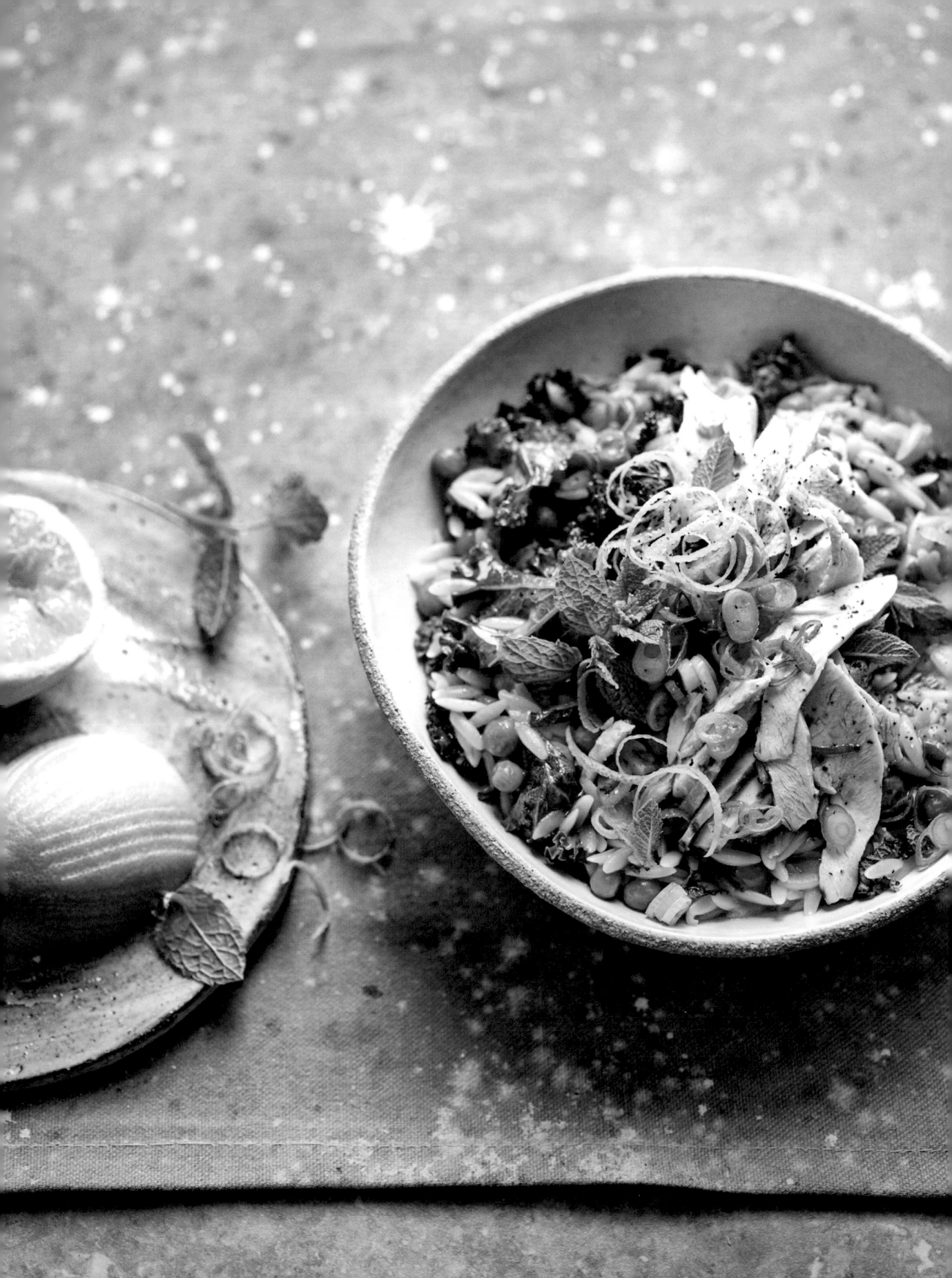

Spiced Potato Cakes with Bacon and Tomato Sauce

This is a such a tasty recipe. I wish there was a photo to show you how good it looks. You'll have to just trust me and go for it.

Ingredients

150g herb-flavoured passata
2 cloves garlic, crushed
salt and pepper
150g midget trees (tenderstem broccoli), sliced thinly
300g cooked potatoes, peeled and roughly mashed
1 red chilli, de-seeded and finely chopped
1 tsp ground cumin
1 tsp ground turmeric
1 tsp curry powder
1 tbsp coriander, chopped
½ tbsp coconut oil
3 lean rashers of bacon (all visible fat removed)

Method

Place the passata and one of the garlic cloves in a small saucepan. Bring to the boil, then reduce the heat and allow to simmer gently for 8–10 minutes. Season and set aside.

Boil the broccoli until just tender, drain and keep warm.

Meanwhile, mix the potatoes with the chilli, cumin, turmeric, curry powder and coriander in a bowl. Using your hands, shape the mixture into three patties.

Preheat the grill to medium-high.

Melt the oil in a large non-stick frying pan and cook the patties for 2–3 minutes on each side, or until lightly browned.

While the cakes are cooking, grill the bacon for 1–2 minutes on each side, or until crisp and lightly golden.

To serve, place the broccoli and the potato cakes on a plate. Drizzle over the tomato sauce and top with bacon.

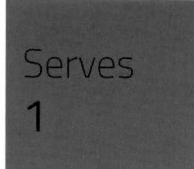

Korean Minced Beef and Quinoa Bowl

This is what Lean in 15 is all about to me. A few ingredients, thrown into a pan, which taste awesome together.

Ingredients

60g quinoa
½ tbsp coconut oil
2 cloves garlic, crushed
½ tsp grated ginger
225g extra-lean steak mince
1 tbsp soy sauce
1 tbsp Korean hot pepper paste
  (gochujang) or hot chilli sauce
2 spring onions, thinly sliced
½ red pepper, de-seeded and
  sliced, for garnish

Method

Cook the quinoa according to packet instructions.

Melt the oil in a non-stick frying pan over a medium heat. Cook the garlic and ginger for about 1 minute, stirring constantly. Add the beef mince and stir-fry until sealed and browned.

In a small bowl, combine the soy sauce and hot pepper paste or chilli sauce.

Add the soy sauce mixture to the beef and stir-fry for 3–5 minutes to allow the flavours to meld.

Place the quinoa in a bowl, top with the beef mixture and sprinkle over the spring onions and red pepper.

Post-workout

Serves
1

Chicken and Vegetable Satay Noodles

This is one for the peanut butter lovers. I love it with noodles but you could also use a bag of cooked rice.

Ingredients

200g chicken mini fillets
2 tbsp soy sauce
1 tsp cornflour
½ tbsp coconut oil
3 spring onions, sliced
1 tbsp smooth peanut butter
1 tbsp sweet chilli sauce
100ml coconut milk
100ml boiling hot
  chicken stock
100g sugarsnap peas, trimmed
50g frozen peas
50g frozen sweetcorn
juice of 1 lime
salt and pepper
200g fresh egg noodles
1 tbsp cashew nuts, chopped
1 tbsp coriander, chopped

Method

Put the chicken in a bowl, add the soy sauce and cornflour and mix well. Cover and set aside for a few moments.

Melt the oil a non-stick frying pan or wok, add the spring onions and stir-fry for 1 minute, or until softened. Add the peanut butter, chilli sauce, coconut milk and stock and stir until combined. Bring to a simmer, then add the marinated chicken and poach for 4–5 minutes, or until cooked through.

Add the sugarsnap peas and simmer for another 2 minutes, or until nearly tender, then add the frozen peas and sweetcorn. Return to the boil, stir in the lime juice and season well.

Stir in the noodles and heat for 1–2 minutes, or until hot through. Serve in a bowl, topped with the cashews and coriander.

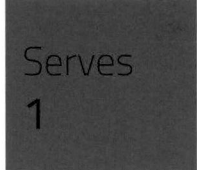

Prosciutto-wrapped Chicken with Corn Mash

Imagine stuffing a chicken breast with sundried tomatoes and wrapping it in ham. Serve it with mashed potato and creamed sweetcorn. Mmmmm. Enjoy.

Ingredients

1 x 180g skinless chicken
   breast fillet
3 sundried tomatoes, chopped
1 slice of prosciutto or
   parma ham
150g potatoes, peeled and cut
   into small pieces
100g green beans, trimmed
100g tinned
   creamed-style corn
1 tbsp chives, finely snipped
salt and pepper

Method

Preheat the oven to 200°C (fan 180°C/gas mark 6). Line a baking tray with baking parchment.

Using a sharp knife, cut a large slit into the side of the chicken breast. Stuff the breast with the sundried tomatoes and wrap the chicken in the prosciutto.

Heat a non-stick frying pan over a high heat and cook the chicken for 1–2 minutes on each side, or until golden. Transfer to the prepared tray and bake for 10–12 minutes, or until cooked through.

Meanwhile, cook the potatoes in a pan of boiling water for 10–12 minutes, or until tender. Steam the green beans.

Drain the potatoes and return to the pan and mash until fairly smooth. Stir in the corn and chives and season well.

Slice the chicken in half and serve with the mash and green beans.

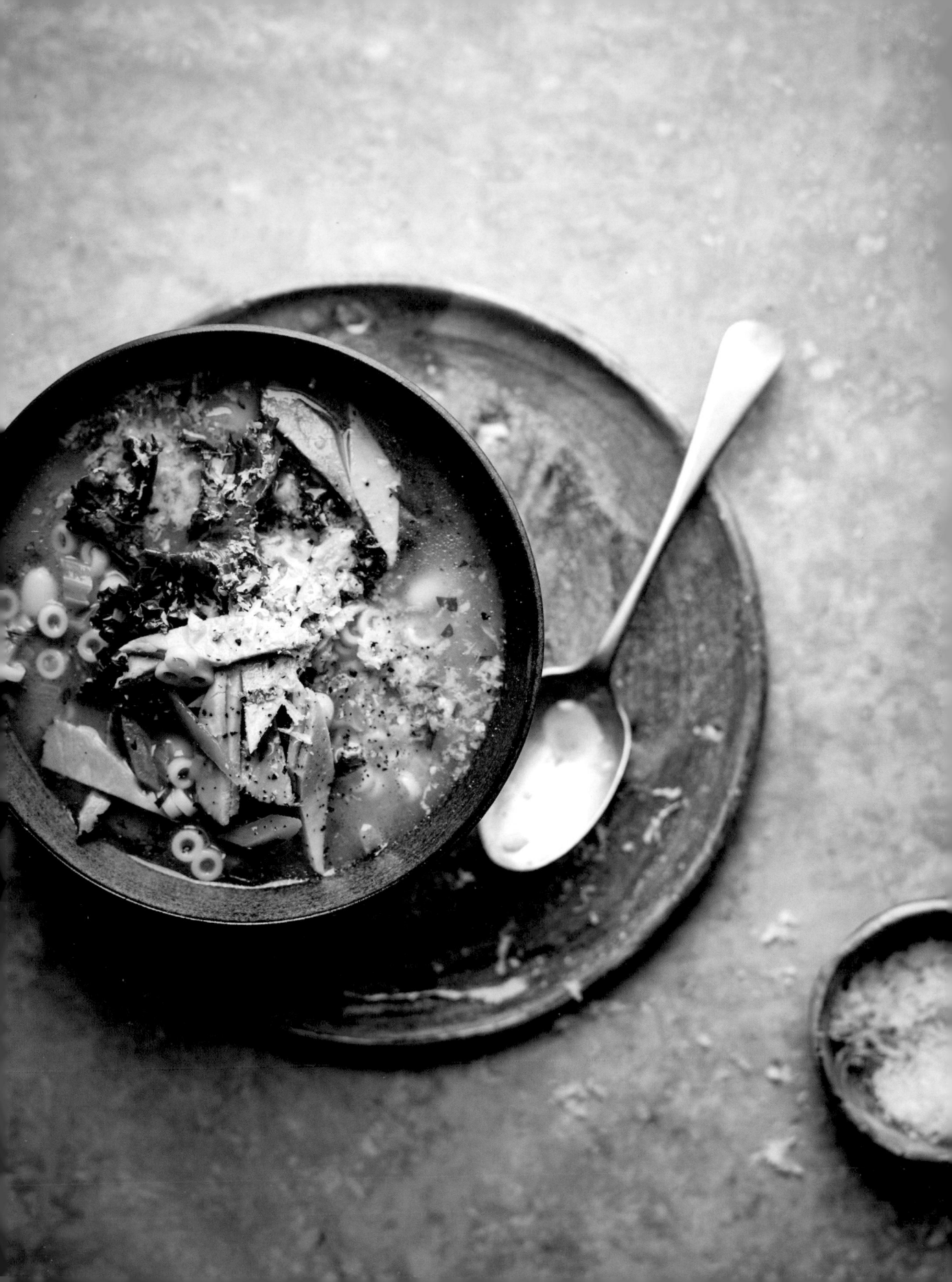

Ham and Bean Minestrone

If you're looking for a hearty soup full of healthy ingredients, this recipe is right up your street. If you don't like ham you could use some shredded pre-cooked chicken breast instead.

Ingredients

½ tbsp coconut oil
½ carrot, finely diced
1 celery stick, finely diced
1 banana shallot, finely diced
1–2 cloves garlic, crushed
pinch of red chilli flakes
100g (drained weight) tinned
  cannellini beans
50g small soup pasta shapes,
  such as orzo or spaghetti,
  broken into small pieces
400ml hot chicken or
  vegetable stock
75g kale, shredded
2 tbsp flat-leaf parsley, chopped
2 slices of deli-style ham, cut
  into thin strips
1 tbsp grated parmesan
  (optional)

Method

Melt the oil in a non-stick frying pan over a medium heat. Add the carrot, celery, shallot, garlic and chilli flakes.

Stir-fry the whole lot for 2–3 minutes, or until softened, then chuck in the beans, pasta and stock. Stir, bring to a simmer and cook for 5–8 minutes, or until the pasta is cooked through.

Stir in the kale, parsley and ham and cook for 1–2 minutes, or until the kale is wilted.

Ladle into a bowl and serve with the parmesan, if using.

Post-workout

Chorizo and Boston Baked Beans with Mash

Next time you wake up craving a greasy fry-up in the cafe, give this recipe a go instead. It's way healthier and tastes much better.

Ingredients

½ tbsp coconut oil
50g chorizo, cut into 1cm pieces
4 spring onions, sliced
½ carrot, very finely diced
1 celery stick, very finely diced
50g onion-and-garlic
   flavoured passata
1 x 220g tin of baked beans
½ tsp mustard powder
4 tbsp tomato puree
½ tbsp balsamic vinegar
½ tbsp dark muscovado sugar
   or honey or black treacle
salt and pepper
150g potatoes, peeled and cut
   into small pieces
1 medium poached or fried egg,
   to serve

Method

Melt the oil in a pan over a medium heat and fry the chorizo and spring onions for 1–2 minutes, until softened.

Add the carrot, celery, passata, baked beans, mustard powder, puree, balsamic and sugar. Bring to the boil then cook at a rolling simmer for 10–12 minutes to thicken and reduce.

Meanwhile, cook the potatoes in a pan of boiling water for 10–12 minutes, or until tender. Drain the potatoes, return to the pan and mash until fairly smooth.

Season the beans and serve with the mash, topped with a poached or fried egg.

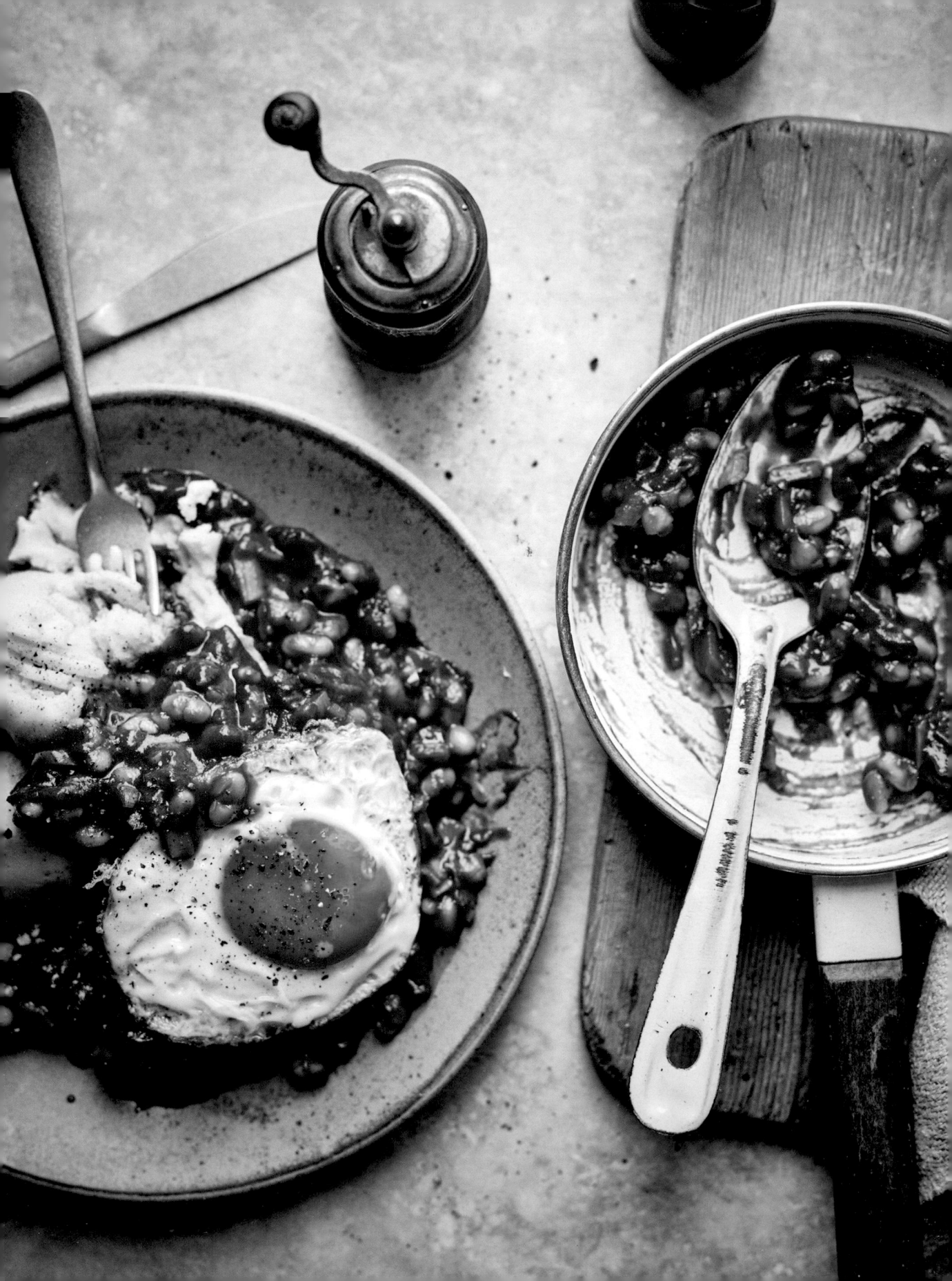

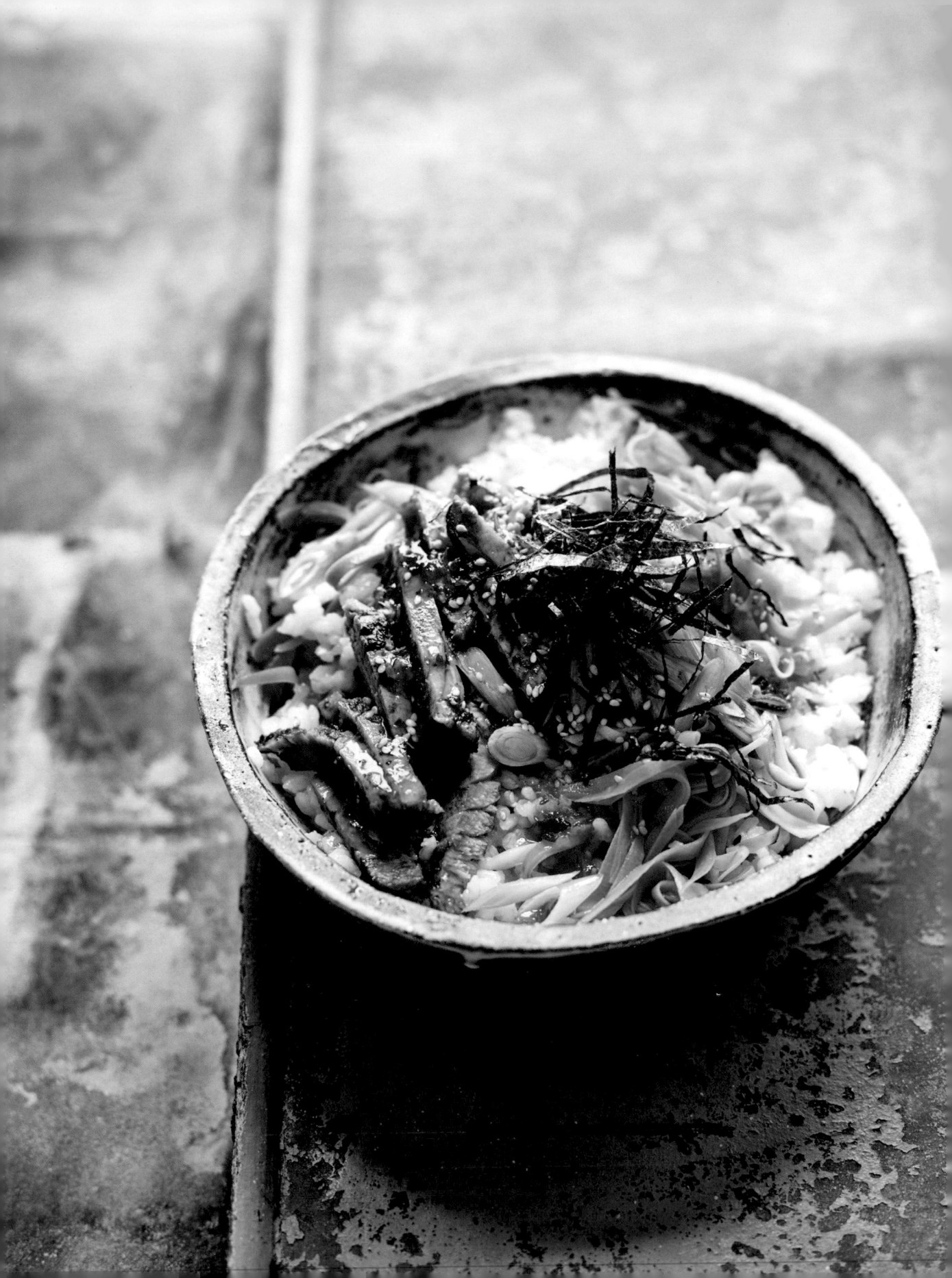

Japanese Sushi Rice Bowl

If you enjoy eating sushi then this recipe is perfect for you. I've used tuna steak here but you could also use chicken breast.

Ingredients

1 x 225g tuna steak
1 tbsp soy sauce
1 clove garlic, crushed
1 tsp grated ginger
black pepper
½ tbsp coconut oil
½ courgette, cut into long
   matchsticks
½ carrot, cut into long
   matchsticks
200g ready-to-eat sushi rice
2 spring onions, very thinly
   sliced
1 tbsp toasted sesame seeds
1 tsp sesame oil
1 tbsp sweet chilli sauce
¼ sheet of nori (seaweed), cut
   into thin strips

Method

Mix the steak with the soy sauce, garlic, ginger and a grind of black pepper.

Melt the oil in a non-stick frying pan. Sear the tuna steak for 1–2 minutes on each side, or until cooked to your liking. Cover and keep warm.

Tip the courgette and carrot into the pan, stir-fry for 1 minute, then push to one side and add the rice. Cook for 1–2 minutes to heat through.

Remove from the heat and toss in the spring onions, half the sesame seeds and sesame oil. Place in a wide bowl.

Thinly slice the tuna and place on top of the rice. Drizzle over the sweet chilli sauce and scatter the nori on top.

Top with the nori and sprinkle over the remaining sesame seeds before serving.

One-Pot Prawn, Vegetable and Lentil Pilaf

This is a perfect example of quick and easy cooking at its best. All in one pot. No messing around, just lots of flavour.

Ingredients

½ tbsp coconut oil
1 tbsp cumin seeds
¼ tsp ground cinnamon
1 red onion, finely sliced
¼ carrot, coarsely grated
¼ courgette, coarsely grated
250g pre-cooked rice
50ml hot vegetable stock
200g (drained weight) tinned
  green lentils, rinsed and
  drained
small handful of baby
  spinach leaves, chopped
200g cooked peeled tiger
  prawns
small handful of
  coriander, chopped
lemon wedges, to serve

Method

Melt the oil in a wide non-stick frying pan over a medium heat and add the cumin seeds, cinnamon, onion, carrot and courgette.

Stir-fry for 3–4 minutes. Add the rice, stock and lentils and stir-fry over a high heat for another 3–4 minutes.

Stir in the spinach and prawns. Cover and cook for 2–3 minutes, or until the prawns are hot and the spinach has wilted. Stir in the coriander and serve with the lemon wedges.

Post-workout

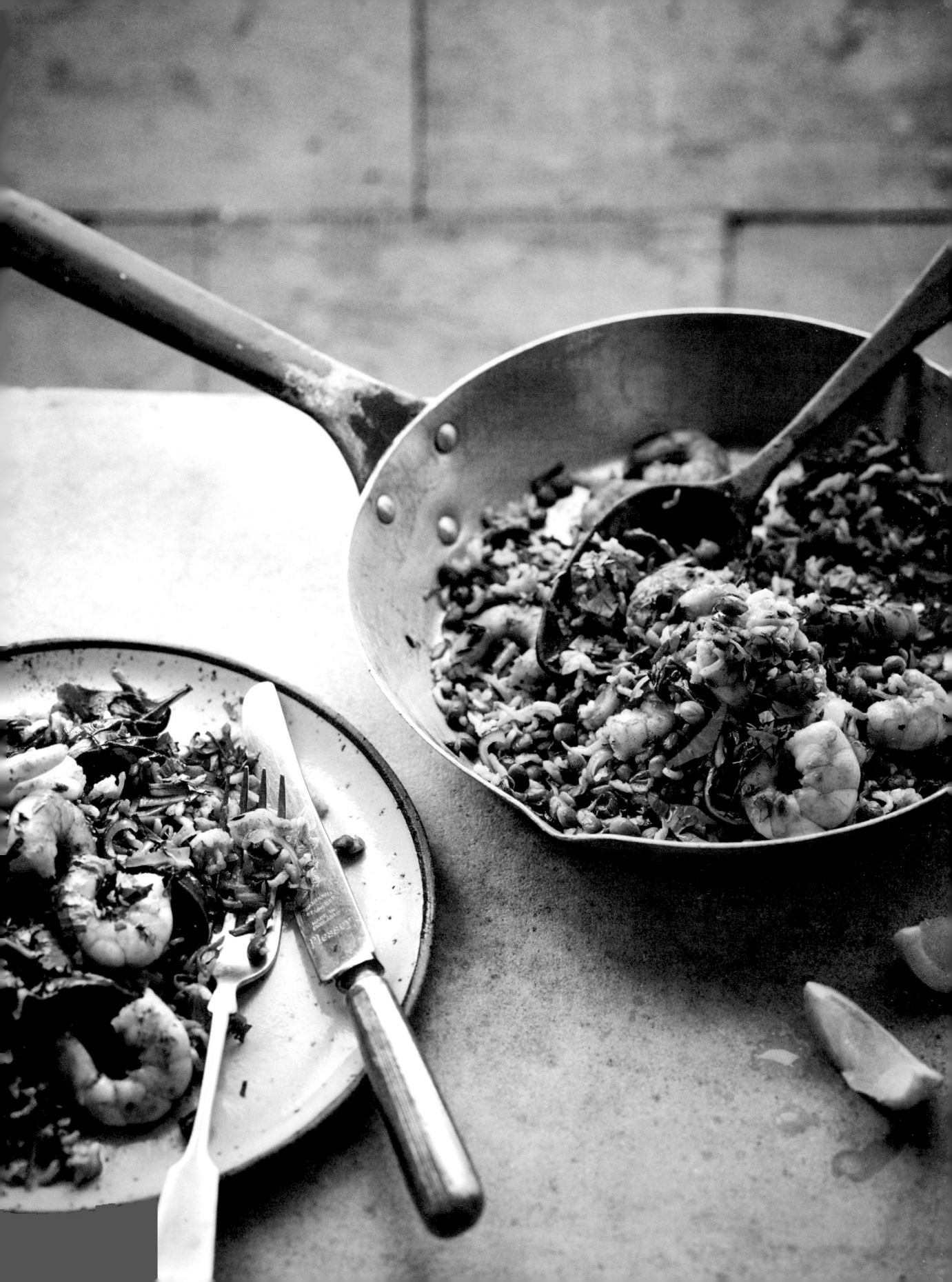

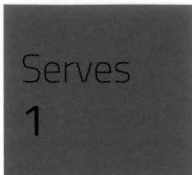
Chicken and Green Pesto Gnocchi

I love every type of pasta but my favourite is probably gnocchi. It's a different texture to normal pasta as it contains potato. If you can't be bothered to make your own pesto, you can also use a ready-made one.

Ingredients

1 x 180g skinless chicken
  breast fillet
½ tbsp coconut oil
200g fresh gnocchi
50g sun-blushed tomatoes,
  drained and roughly chopped
30g grilled artichoke hearts,
  drained and roughly chopped
small handful of wild rocket
  leaves, roughly chopped

For the pesto

large handful of basil leaves
  (about 50g), finely chopped
1–2 cloves garlic, crushed
2 tbsp half-fat crème fraiche
1 tsp finely grated lemon zest
1 red chilli, de-seeded and
  chopped
salt and pepper

Method

Place the chicken between two pieces of cling film, and using a rolling pin or wooden mallet, lightly beat until slightly thinned to an even thickness.

Melt the coconut oil on a hot griddle pan and cook the chicken for 6–8 minutes on each side, until cooked through. Check by slicing into it to make sure the meat is white all the way through, with no raw pink bits left. Set aside.

Meanwhile, cook the gnocchi according to packet instructions.

Make the pesto by placing all the ingredients in a small food processor and blitzing until fairly smooth. Season and set aside.

Shred the cooked chicken. Place the tomatoes, artichokes, chicken, rocket and cooked gnocchi in a bowl. Pour over the pesto and toss to mix well. Eat immediately or at room temperature.

Post-workout

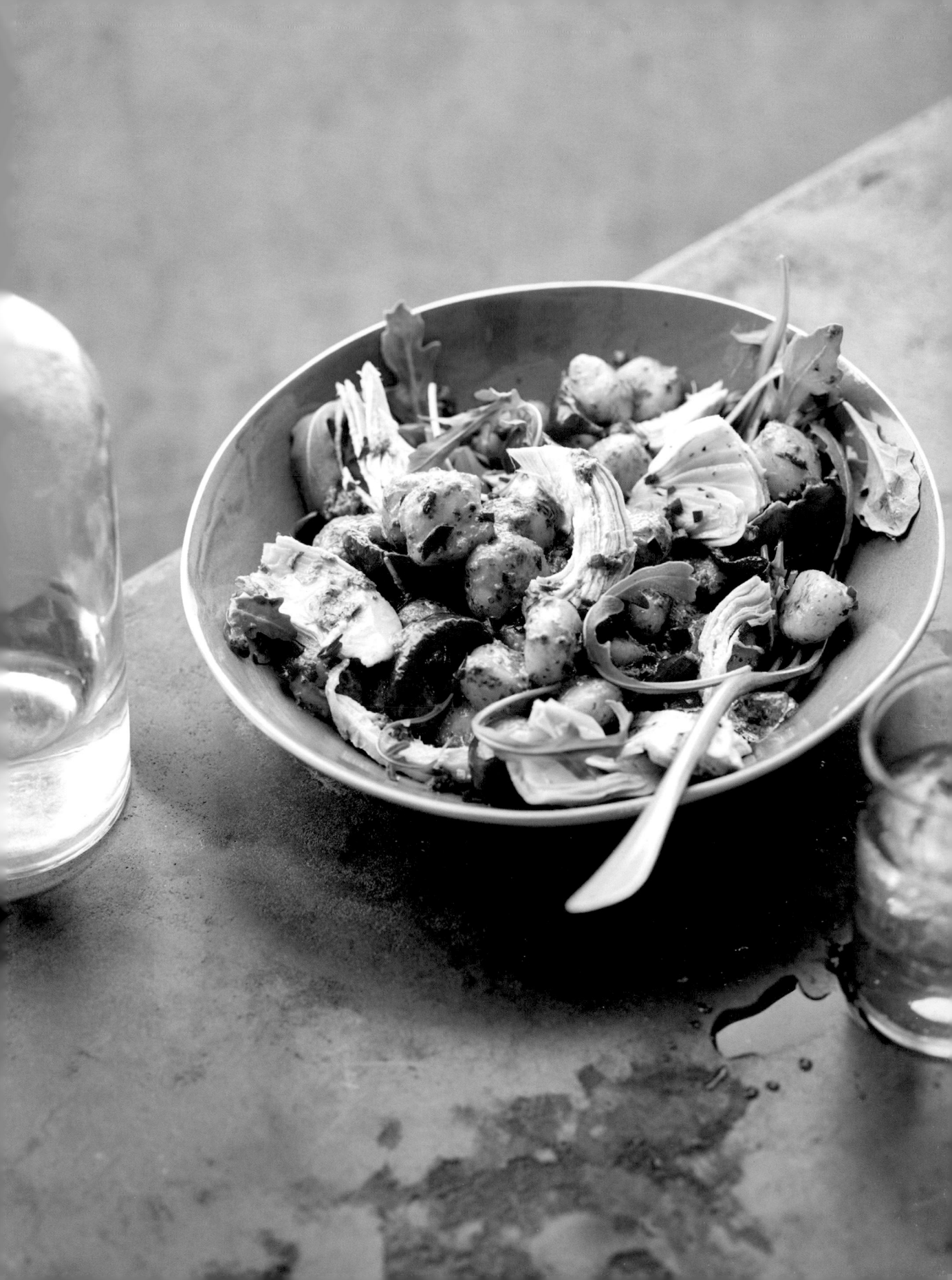

Mango Chicken Burger

I'm back with another burger recipe and I'm going to say I think this is my best one ever. Just stare at that photo for a few moments. I hope you love making it as much as I do.

Ingredients

1 large sweet potato
½ tbsp coconut oil
salt and pepper
1 x 180g skinless chicken breast fillet, roughly chopped
1 tsp grated ginger
1 tsp grated garlic
1 red chilli, chopped – remove the seeds if you don't like it hot
2 tbsp coriander, chopped
1 tbsp mint, chopped
zest and juice of ½ lime
1 slice of white bread, crumbed

To serve

1 tbsp zero-fat Greek-style yoghurt
large brioche bun, split in half and toasted
2 gem lettuce leaves, roughly torn, plus extra for side salad
2–3 slices of tomato
3–4 cucumber ribbons, sliced with a vegetable peeler
1 tbsp mango chutney

Method

To make the sweet potato chips, preheat the oven to 200°C (fan 180°C/gas mark 6). Cut the large sweet potato into chips and toss them with the coconut oil. Season with salt and pepper. Roast in the oven for 12–15 minutes, until lightly browned.

Meanwhile, place the chicken, ginger, garlic, chilli, coriander, zest and juice and breadcrumbs into a food processor. Season and blitz until well blended.

Preheat the grill to medium.

Shape the mixture into a large patty and place under the grill for 5–6 minutes on each side, or until cooked through and lightly golden.

To serve, spread the yoghurt on the base half of the toasted brioche bun. Top with the lettuce, tomato and cucumber ribbons.

Place the burger on top, spread over the mango chutney and top with the toasted bun lid. Serve with the sweet potato chips.

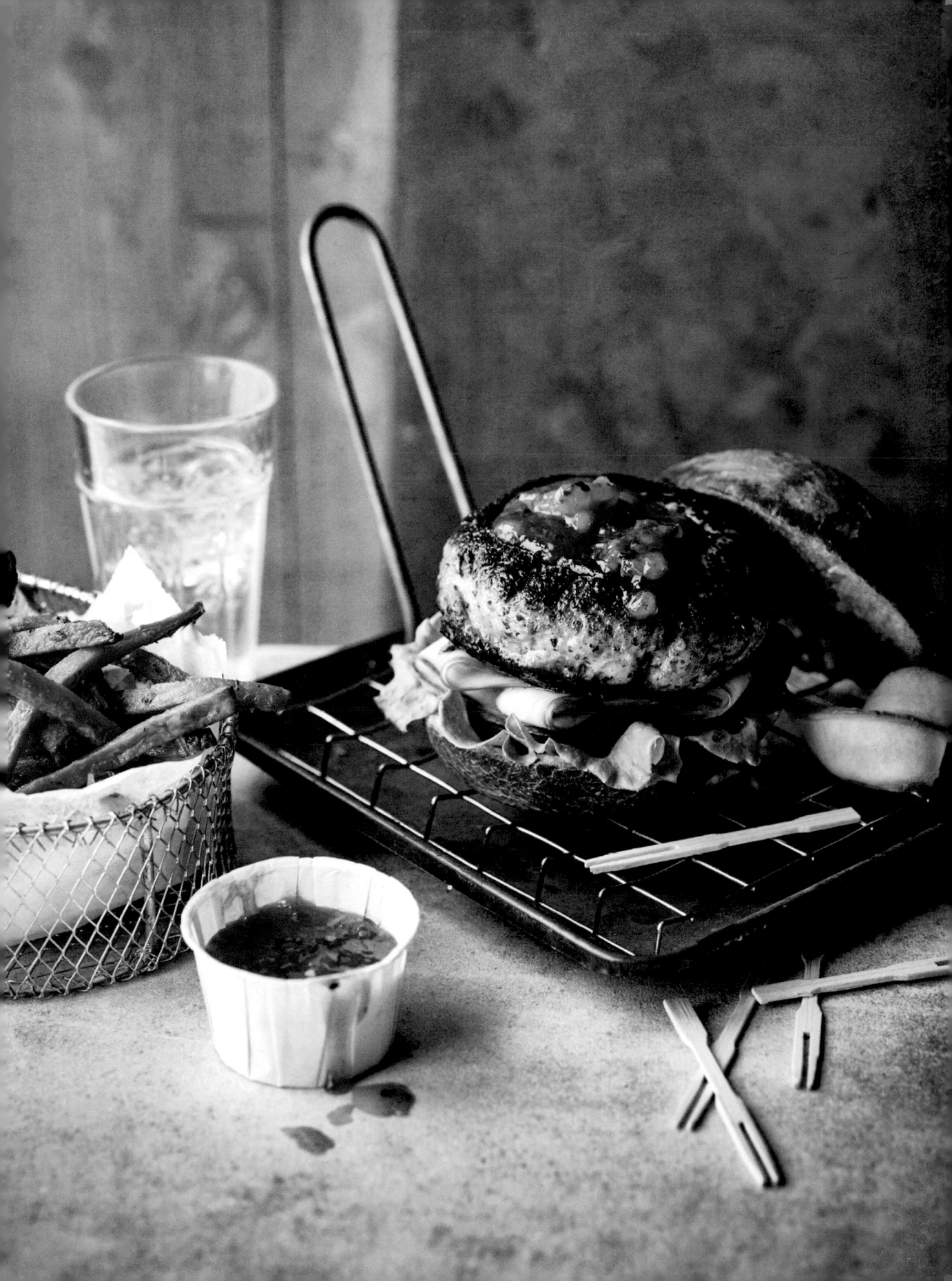

Sweet and Spicy Steak and Noodle Salad

Fresh flavours and healthy ingredients make this recipe one not to be missed. It's a lean taste of Asia that I think you'll love.

Ingredients

2 tbsp light soy sauce
1 tsp finely grated garlic
1 tsp finely grated ginger
1 lean fillet or sirloin steak
250g cooked rice noodles
¼ carrot, finely julienned
   or grated
½ red pepper, de-seeded and
   very thinly sliced
2 spring onions, finely
   shredded
1 tbsp mint, finely chopped,
   plus extra sprigs for garnish
2 tbsp coriander, chopped
   (optional)
½ tbsp toasted sesame seeds
½ red chilli, very thinly sliced
   – remove the seeds if you
   don't like it hot

For the dressing

1 tbsp mirin
1 tbsp dark soy sauce
¼ tsp sesame oil
1 tbsp sweet chilli sauce
1 tsp finely grated ginger

Method

Make the marinade by placing the soy sauce, garlic and ginger in a bowl, and mix well.

Put the steak in a shallow dish and spoon the marinade over both sides. Leave to marinate for 5 minutes, or longer if you have the time.

Heat a griddle pan until hot over a high heat. Pat the steaks dry with kitchen roll and sear for about 2 minutes on each side for medium rare. Give the meat another minute or so if you prefer it well done. Transfer to a board, cut into thin strips and set aside.

Combine all the dressing ingredients together in a small bowl.

Place the noodles in a colander and refresh with cold water before transferring to a bowl. Combine the noodles with the dressing to coat well.

Mix the carrot, pepper, spring onions, mint, coriander (if using) and sesame seeds with the noodles.

Spoon into a bowl and top with the sliced beef fillet and juices. Sprinkle with extra mint and red chilli.

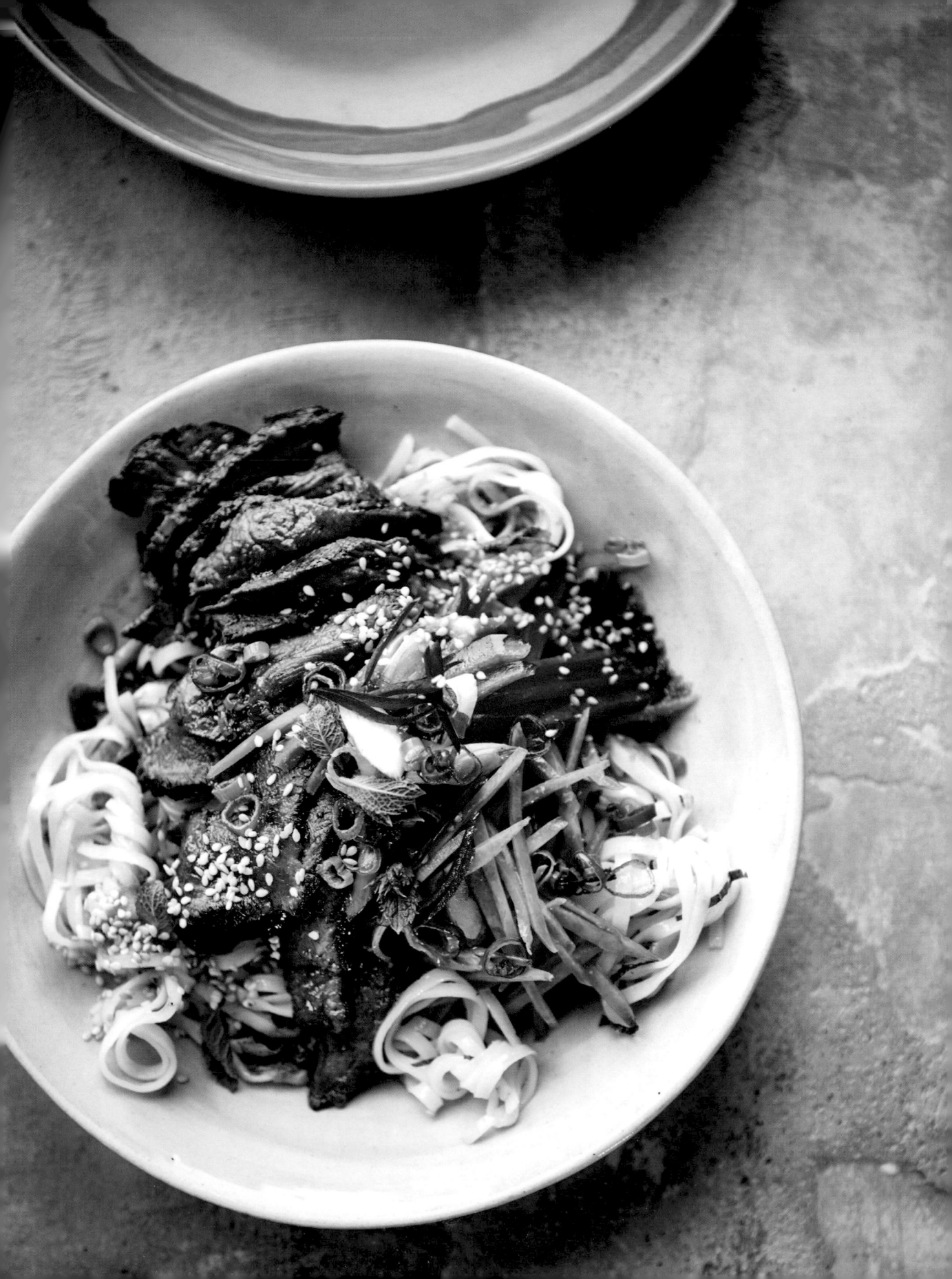

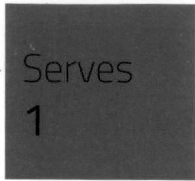

Pork Arrabbiata with Spaghetti

My Grandma Carmela is Italian, so this is another recipe inspired by her. I think Italian food is some of the best in the world: simple yet always so full of flavour.

Ingredients

95g spaghetti
½ tbsp coconut oil
1 x 200g lean pork tenderloin fillet, very thinly sliced
2–3 anchovies in oil, drained and chopped
2 cloves garlic, crushed
¼ tsp dried red chilli flakes
2 ripe plum tomatoes, finely chopped (about 200–250g)
2 tbsp flat-leaf parsley, chopped
20g pitted kalamata olives
salt and pepper
1 tbsp oregano, chopped

Method

Cook the spaghetti according to packet instructions. Drain thoroughly.

Meanwhile, melt the oil in a wide non-stick frying pan over a high heat. Add the pork slices and cook for 2 minutes on each side until cooked through and browned. Transfer to a plate with a slotted spoon and keep warm.

Chuck the anchovies, garlic and chilli into the pan and stir for 30 seconds. Add the tomatoes and cook over a medium heat for 8–10 minutes, stirring occasionally, until the sauce has reduced and thickened.

Stir in the parsley and olives and heat for 1–2 minutes. Season.

Add the spaghetti to the pan and toss to coat evenly. Transfer to a plate, top with the pork and sprinkle over the oregano before serving.

Asian-spiced Mi
Beef Noodle Bo

If you want to prep like a boss, double this recipe – you can have half today and half for lunch at work tomorrow. Just reheat in the microwave for a few minutes.

Ingredients

½ tbsp coconut oil

¼ tsp dried red chilli flakes

¼ tsp crushed Szechuan peppercorns

200g extra-lean steak mince

4 spring onions, white and green parts separated and thinly sliced

2 tbsp light soy sauce

½ tbsp Shaoxing rice wine

1 tbsp sweet chilli sauce

¼ tsp sesame oil

200g cooked medium egg noodles

1 fried medium egg (optional)

1 tbsp roasted peanuts, roughly chopped

Method

Melt the oil in large non-stick frying pan. Add the chilli and Szechuan peppercorns and cook gently for 3–4 minutes, allowing the flavours to meld into the oil.

Slide in the beef mince and spring onion whites. Cook, turning up the heat and letting the mince brown really well (you want to get some browned crispy bits on it). Stir in half the soy sauce and keep warm.

Mix the rest of the soy, rice wine, sweet chilli sauce and sesame oil and toss with the cooked noodles. Top with the beef mix, spring onion greens and the fried egg (if using) and scatter over the peanuts just before serving.

Post-workout

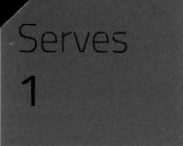
Lemon and Dill Salmon Burgers with Caper Dressing

The flavours in these burgers and dressing are outrageous. I think you will love this and make it over and over again.

Ingredients

1 thick slice of white bread

1 x 200g skinless, boneless salmon fillet

2 spring onions, finely chopped

1 tbsp dill, chopped, plus extra for garnish

2 tsp finely grated lemon zest

pinch of dried red chilli flakes

1 small egg white

salt and pepper

½ tbsp coconut oil

100g midget trees (tenderstem broccoli), thinly sliced lengthways

200g pre-cooked basmati rice, to serve

salt and black pepper

lemon wedges, to serve

For the caper gremolata

1 tbsp grated lemon zest

1 clove garlic, very finely diced

2 tbsp flat-leaf parsley, finely chopped

1 tbsp capers

1 tbsp lemon juice

Method

Preheat the oven to 200°C (fan 180°C/gas mark 6). Line a baking tray with baking parchment.

In a food processor, whizz the bread into crumbs. Cut the salmon into chunks, and add it to the processor with the spring onions, dill, lemon zest, chilli flakes and egg white and blitz until just combined.

Season the salmon mixture well and divide into two portions. Shape each into a burger.

Melt the oil in a large non-stick frying pan over a high heat. Brown the burgers for 1 minute on each side, then add to the prepared baking tray and bake for 10 minutes, or until cooked through.

While the salmon is cooking, make the gremolata by mixing together the lemon zest, garlic and parsley. Place in a bowl with the capers and lemon juice. Season well.

Blanch the broccoli in boiling water for 2–3 minutes or until just tender, then drain and add to the cooked rice. Season and toss to mix well.

Serve the salmon burgers over the rice and broccoli mixture and spoon the caper gremolata over the top. Serve with lemon wedges and sprigs of dill.

Post-workout

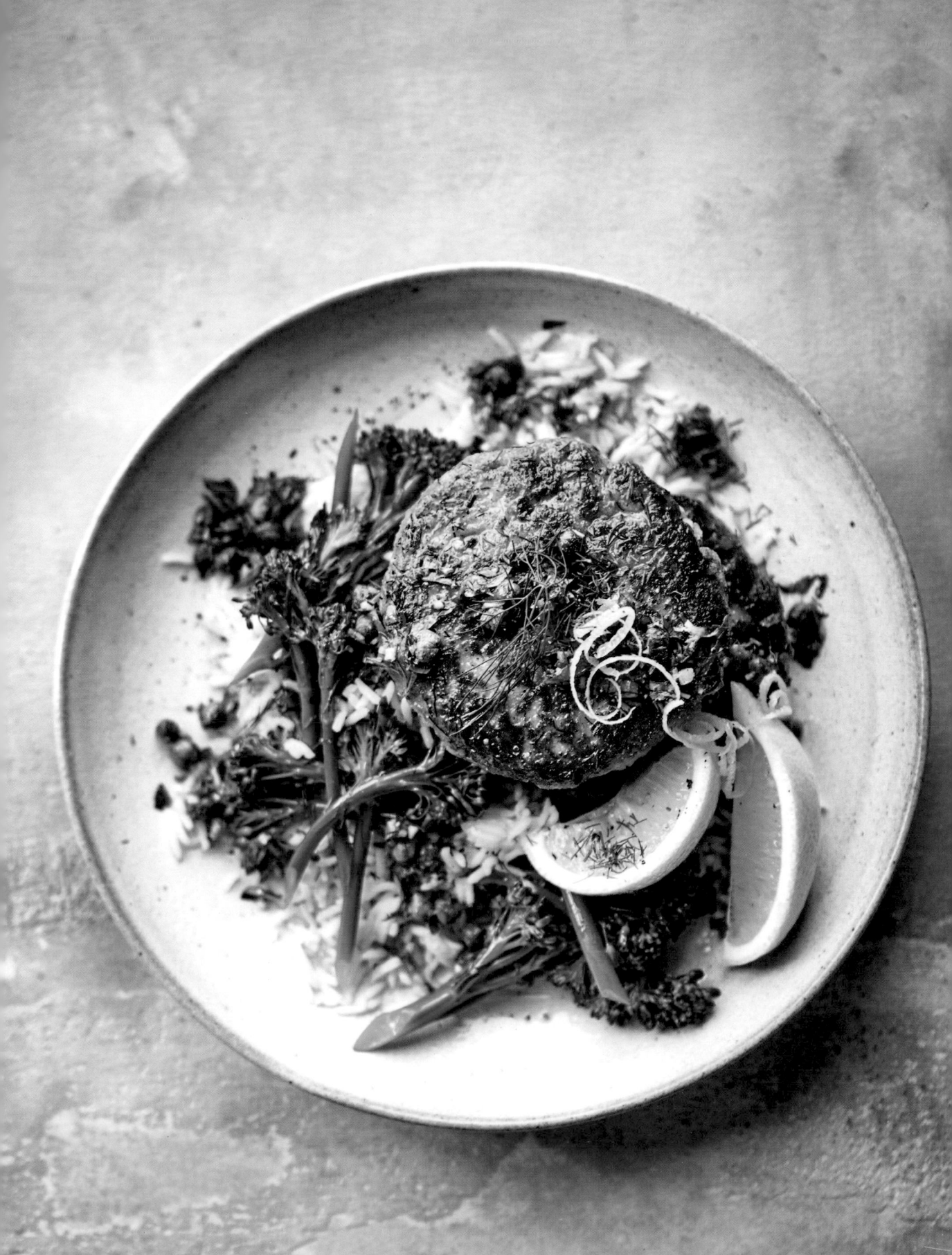

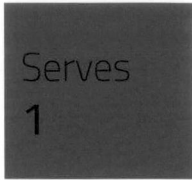

Serves
1

Make ahead

Lemon Rice Salad with Tuna and Green Beans

This is a salad full of flavour that I like to eat after a workout. It can be carried in a lunch box and eaten on the move, too.

Ingredients

1 x 200g pack of pre-cooked brown basmati and wild rice blend
100g green beans, trimmed and halved
½ cucumber, quartered lengthways and sliced
2 shallots, thinly sliced
100g mixed cherry tomatoes, halved
200g (drained weight) tinned tuna in spring water, flaked
20g pitted stuffed green olives
25g flat-leaf parsley, chopped
finely grated lemon zest and juice of 1 lemon
1 red chilli, de-seeded and finely diced (optional)
1 clove garlic, crushed
½ tbsp olive oil
black pepper

Method

Heat the rice according to packet instructions, then transfer to a large bowl and set aside.

Meanwhile, bring a medium saucepan of water to the boil, then blanch the green beans for 2 minutes, or until just tender. Drain the beans, then refresh in a bowl of cold water and pat dry with kitchen roll.

Add the blanched green beans to the rice with the cucumber, shallots, tomatoes, tuna, olives and parsley.

Mix the lemon zest and juice, chilli (if using), garlic and olive oil together in a small bowl to make a dressing, then season with black pepper. Toss through the salad, then serve.

Post-workout

Moroccan Fish with Mango Couscous

The sweetness in this couscous works perfectly with the spicy fish. Quick-cook couscous makes life easy, too.

Ingredients

65g couscous
1 orange
2 tsp Moroccan spice mix
1 tsp runny honey
1 x 225g skinless white
  fish fillet (cod or halibut)
salt and pepper

For the dressing

1 tbsp apple cider vinegar
½ tbsp olive oil
2 tbsp toasted pine nuts
200g diced mango flesh
small handful of chopped
  mint leaves, plus extra
  for garnish

Method

Cook the couscous according to packet instructions.

Zest the orange. Combine the spice mix, honey and orange zest in a small bowl.

Place the fish on a plate and spoon over the spice mix. Season well.

Place the couscous with all the dressing ingredients and the juice and segments from the orange into a bowl. Toss to mix well.

Preheat the grill to medium-high. Place the fish on a grill rack and cook under the grill for 8–10 minutes, or until cooked through.

Plate the couscous mixture onto a plate and top with the grilled fish. Scatter over extra mint and serve.

Quick Chicken, Chorizo and Prawn Spanish Rice

Yum! All my favourite things in one dish. This is a proper, satisfying refuel meal after a workout.

Ingredients

½ x 200g skinless chicken
  breast fillet
1 tbsp coconut oil
100g fine green beans, halved
50g chorizo sausage,
  thinly sliced
2 banana shallots, sliced
1 clove garlic, crushed
250g pre-cooked white or
  basmati rice
50ml boiling hot chicken stock
large pinch of saffron strands
  (or 1 large pinch of ground
  turmeric)
¼ tsp sweet smoked paprika
1 jarred red pepper,
  drained and roughly chopped
100g cooked peeled tiger
  prawns
salt and pepper
2 tbsp flat-leaf parsley,
  finely chopped
slices of lemon, to serve

Method

Place the chicken between two pieces of cling film, and using a rolling pin or wooden mallet, lightly beat until slightly thinned to an even thickness.

Melt ½ tablespoon of the coconut oil on a hot griddle pan and cook the chicken for 6–8 minutes on each side, until cooked through. Check by slicing into it to make sure the meat is white all the way through, with no raw pink bits left. Set aside.

Meanwhile, blanch the green beans in boiling water for 1–2 minutes or until just tender. Drain and keep warm.

Melt the remaining oil in a wide non-stick frying pan and add the chorizo and shallots. Stir-fry for 2–3 minutes, then stir in the garlic and cook for 30 seconds more.

Stir in the rice, boiling hot stock, saffron and paprika and cook over a high heat for 2–3 minutes, until piping hot.

Cut the cooked chicken into 1.5cm dice. Stir in the red pepper, prawns and chicken and stir and cook for 2–3 minutes, or until warmed through.

Remove from the heat, season and stir through the chopped parsley. Serve immediately, with the slices of lemon.

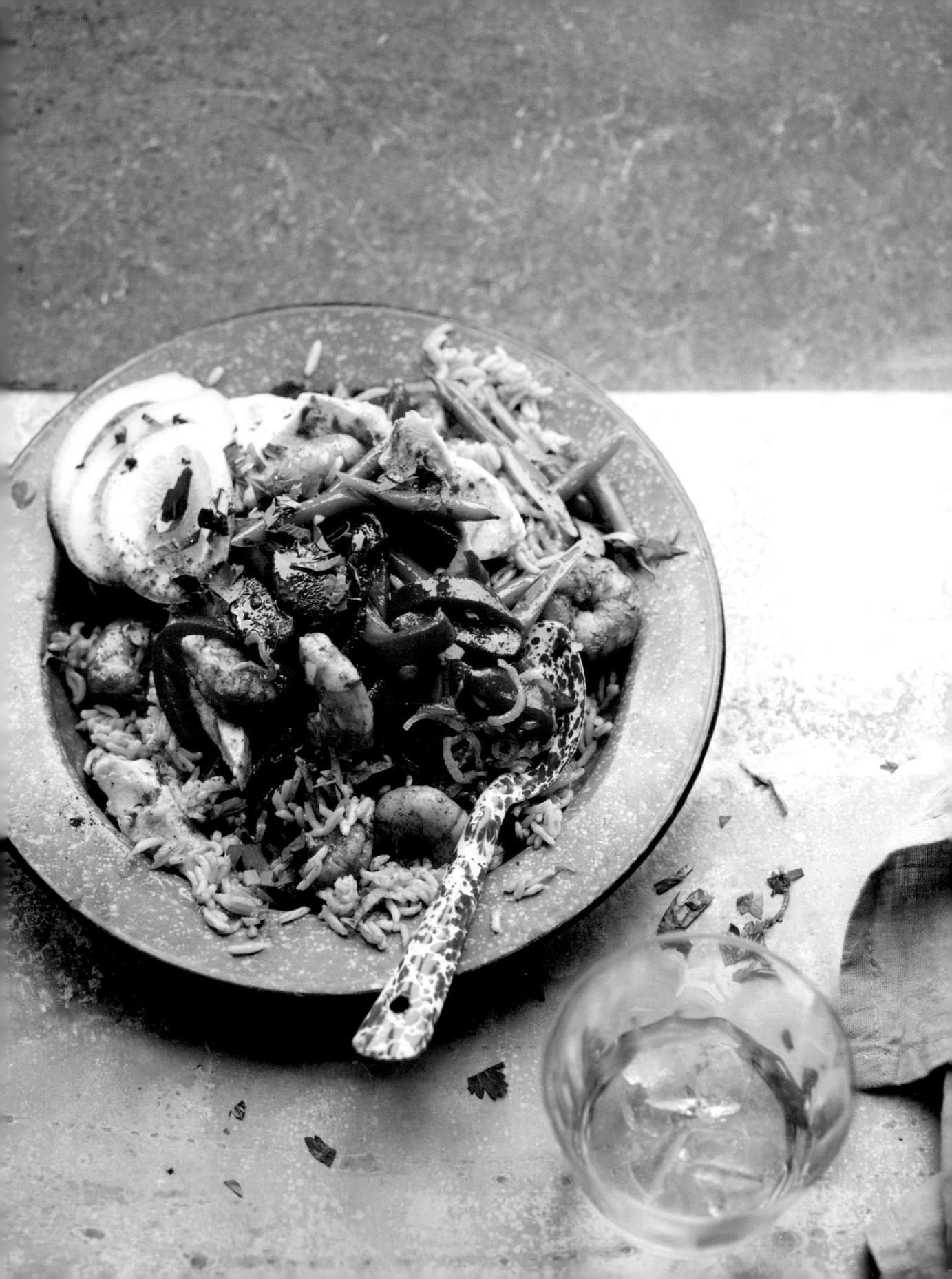

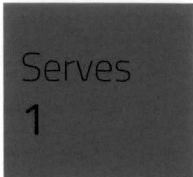

Prawn and Red Curry Noodle Bowl

I'm really proud of this recipe. I hope you give it a go because it tastes unbelievable. You'll definitely make it again.

Ingredients

½ tbsp coconut oil
1–2 tbsp Thai red curry paste (depending on how strong or mild you like it)
200ml coconut milk
100ml vegetable or chicken stock
¼ carrot, cut into thin matchsticks
50g sugarsnap peas, thinly sliced lengthways
1 spring onion, very thinly sliced
½ tsp fish sauce
salt and pepper
200g cooked rice noodles
200g cooked peeled tiger prawns
2 tbsp coriander, chopped
lime wedges, to serve

Method

Melt the oil in a wide non-stick saucepan and add the curry paste. Stir and cook for 30 seconds, then stir in the coconut milk and stock and bring to the boil.

Add the carrot, sugarsnap peas and spring onion and bring back to the boil. Cook for 1 minute.

Add the fish sauce and season. Toss in the noodles and prawns and cook for a further 2–3 minutes until warmed through.

Remove the pan from the heat and transfer to a bowl. Sprinkle over the coriander and squeeze over the wedges of lime.

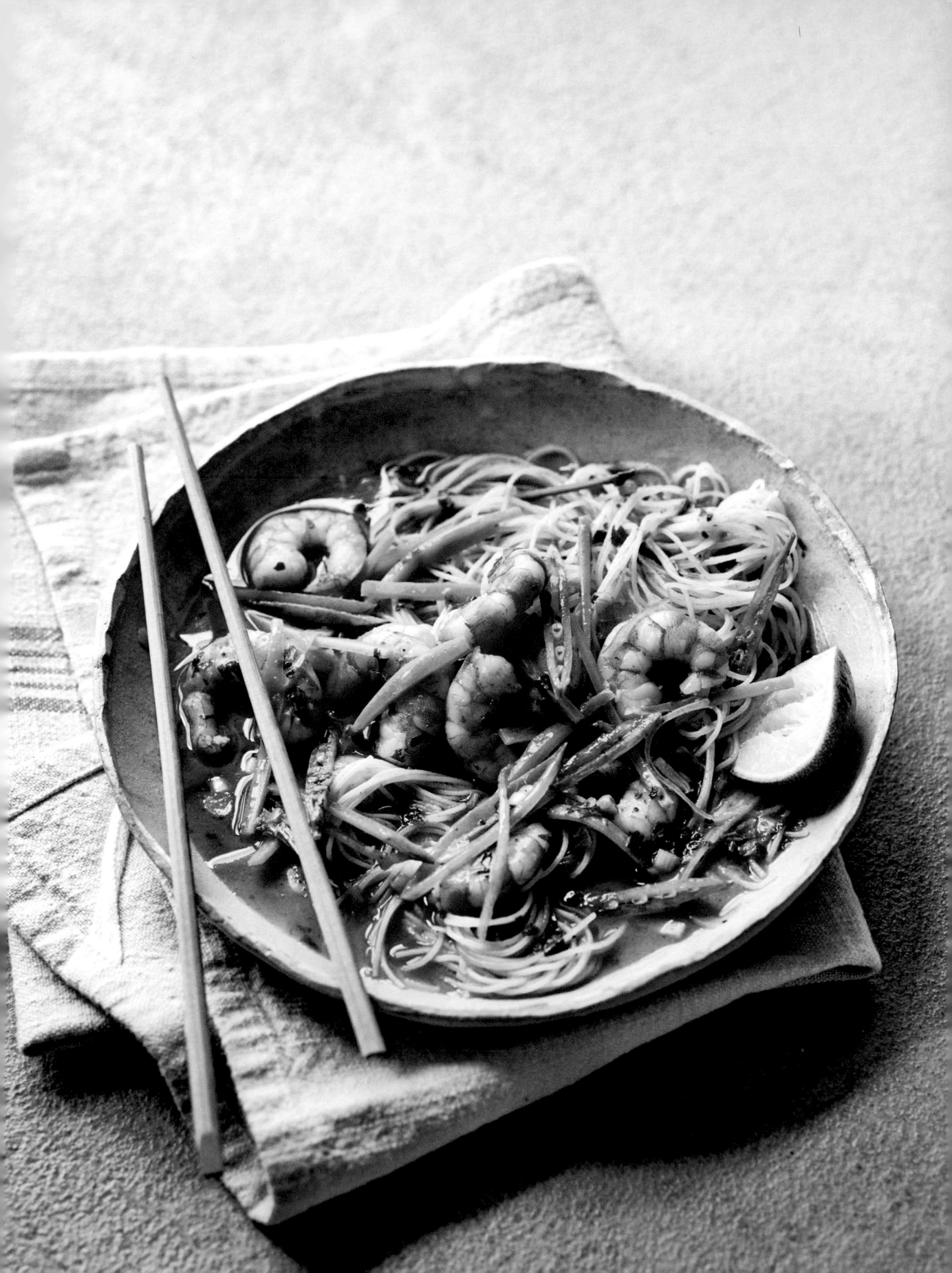

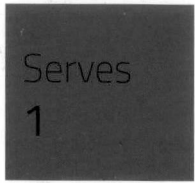

Serves
1

Make ahead

Pancetta Gnocchi with Ham and Rocket

Carbs are not the enemy. This recipe will leave you feeling very satisfied: just the feeling you want after a workout!

Ingredients

200g fresh gnocchi
½ tbsp coconut oil
2 slices of pancetta, roughly chopped
1 small onion, finely chopped
1 clove garlic, crushed
1 red chilli, finely chopped – remove the seeds if you don't like it hot
1 tbsp apple cider vinegar
3 plum tomatoes, finely chopped
salt and pepper
200g thick deli-style ham, roughly chopped
small handful of wild rocket

Method

Cook the gnocchi according to packet instructions.

Melt the oil in a wide non-stick frying pan. Add the pancetta, onion, garlic and chilli and stir-fry for 1–2 minutes.

Stir in the vinegar and tomatoes and simmer for 10 minutes, or until the tomatoes break down and turn mushy, adding a splash of water if needed. Season and stir in the ham, gnocchi and rocket.

Toss to mix well and heat for 1–2 minutes, or until piping hot.

Post-workout

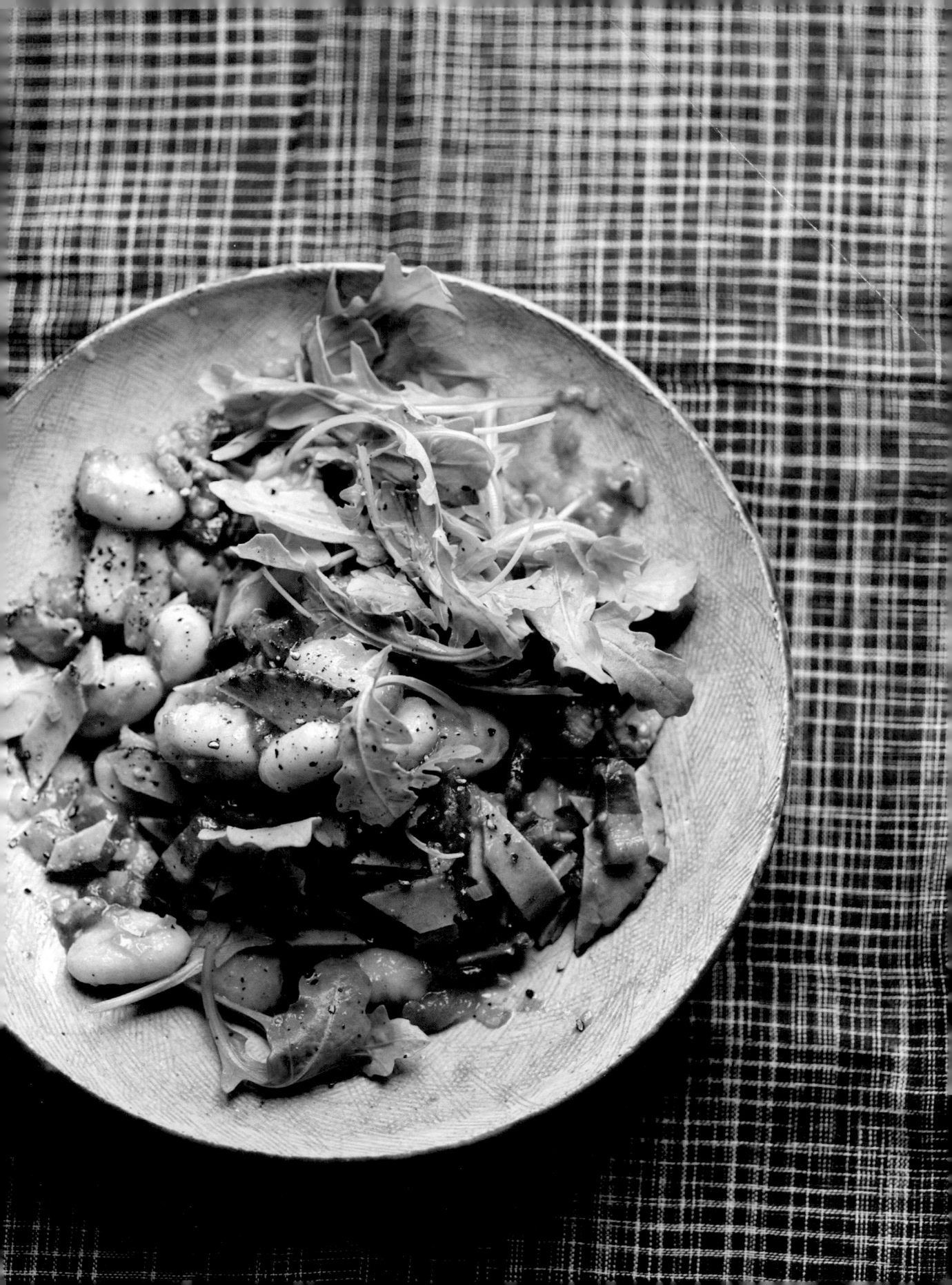

Serves
1

⏱ Make ahead

Ingredients

½ jarred red pepper,
  drained and finely chopped
½ small onion, finely diced
1 red chilli, de-seeded and
  finely diced
1 plum tomato, de-seeded and
  finely diced
finely grated zest of ½ lime
  and the juice of 1 lime
2 tbsp finely chopped
  coriander, plus extra
  for garnish
salt and pepper
1 lean sirloin steak (trimmed
  of all visible fat)
1 tsp cumin seeds
1 tsp coconut oil
2 corn tortillas
handful of shredded iceberg
  lettuce
1 tbsp zero-fat Greek-style
  yoghurt (optional)

Steak Taco with Lime Salsa

Oh, for the love of tacos! Look at that. Wow. This is my dream post-workout meal.

Method

Make the salsa by combining the red pepper, onion, chilli, tomato, lime zest and juice and coriander. Season well and set aside.

Preheat the oven to 180°C (fan 160°C/gas mark 4).

Season the steak and sprinkle with the cumin seeds.

Melt the coconut oil in a non-stick frying pan and sear the steaks, turning once, for 3 minutes each side (for medium rare).

While the steak is cooking, heat the tortilla wraps in the oven for 5 minutes or warm them on a preheated non-stick ridged griddle pan.

To serve, slice the steak into 5mm strips. Place some lettuce leaves down the centre of each tortilla, top with strips of steak, then spoon over the lime salsa. Top with the yoghurt, if using, and roll up. Serve or pack in your lunchbox for later on.

Post-workout

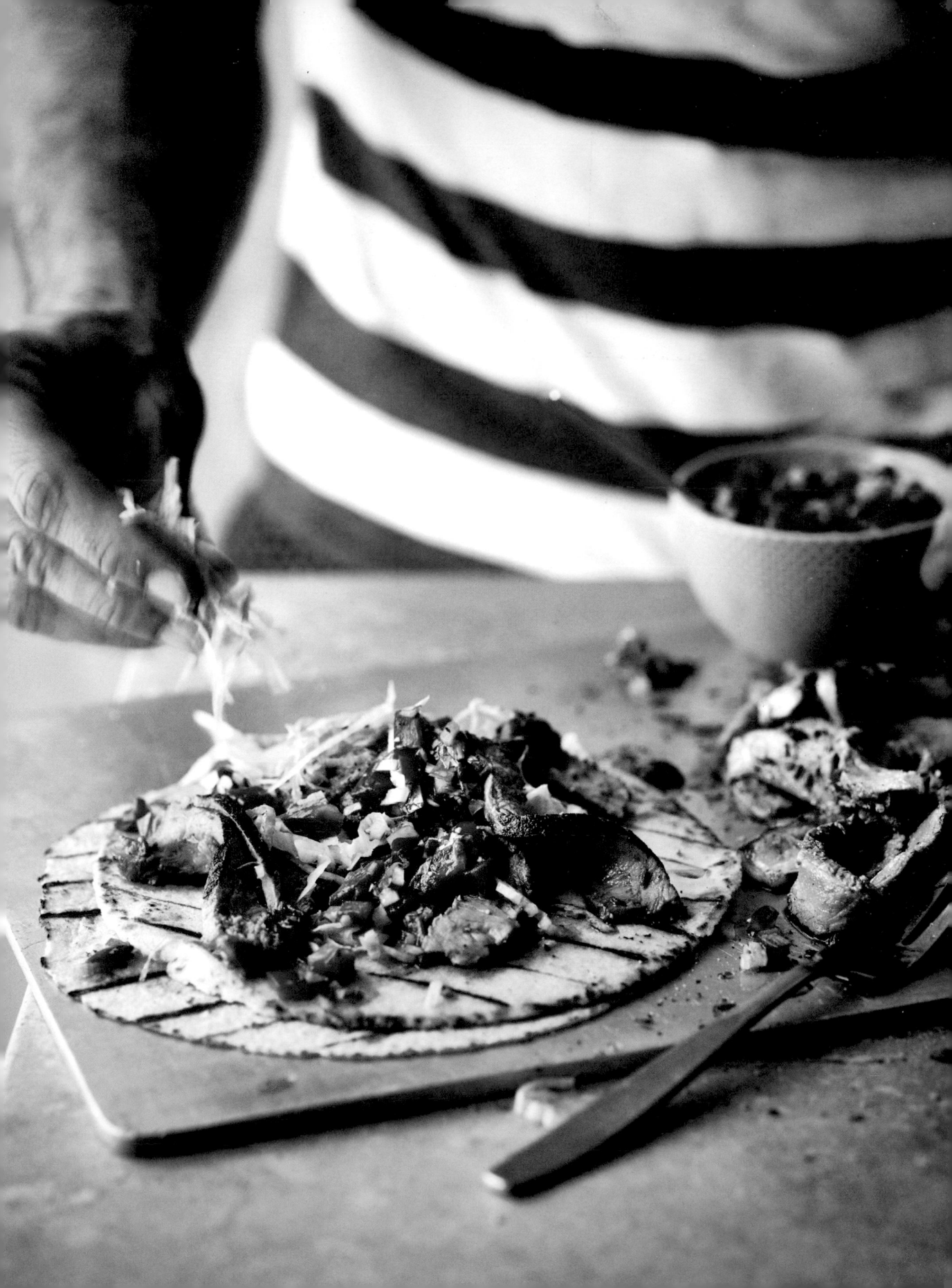

Cheeky Chinese Noodles with Prawns

When you fancy ordering in a Chinese take-away, give this healthy option a go instead.

Ingredients

1 tbsp dark soy sauce

1 tsp fish sauce

3 tbsp oyster sauce

½ tbsp coconut oil

3 spring onions, cut into 2cm diagonal lengths

2 cloves garlic, crushed

1 red chilli, de-seeded and finely chopped

200g raw peeled tiger prawns

4 shiitake mushrooms, sliced

50g midget trees (tenderstem broccoli), thinly sliced lengthways

2–3 baby pak choi, halved or quartered if large (or roughly chopped)

250g cooked rice noodles

Method

Mix the soy sauce, fish sauce and oyster sauce in a bowl and set aside.

Melt the oil in a large non-stick frying pan over a medium heat. Add the spring onions, garlic and the chilli and stir-fry for 20 seconds.

Chuck in the prawns, shiitake mushrooms and broccoli. Stir-fry for 2–3 minutes, then add the pak choi and the sauce mixture. Stir and cook for about 2–3 minutes over a high heat, until the prawns turn pink and are cooked through, adding a splash of water if the sauce becomes too thick.

Stir in the noodles, remove from the heat and toss to mix well. Serve in a warmed bowl and tuck in with your chopsticks.

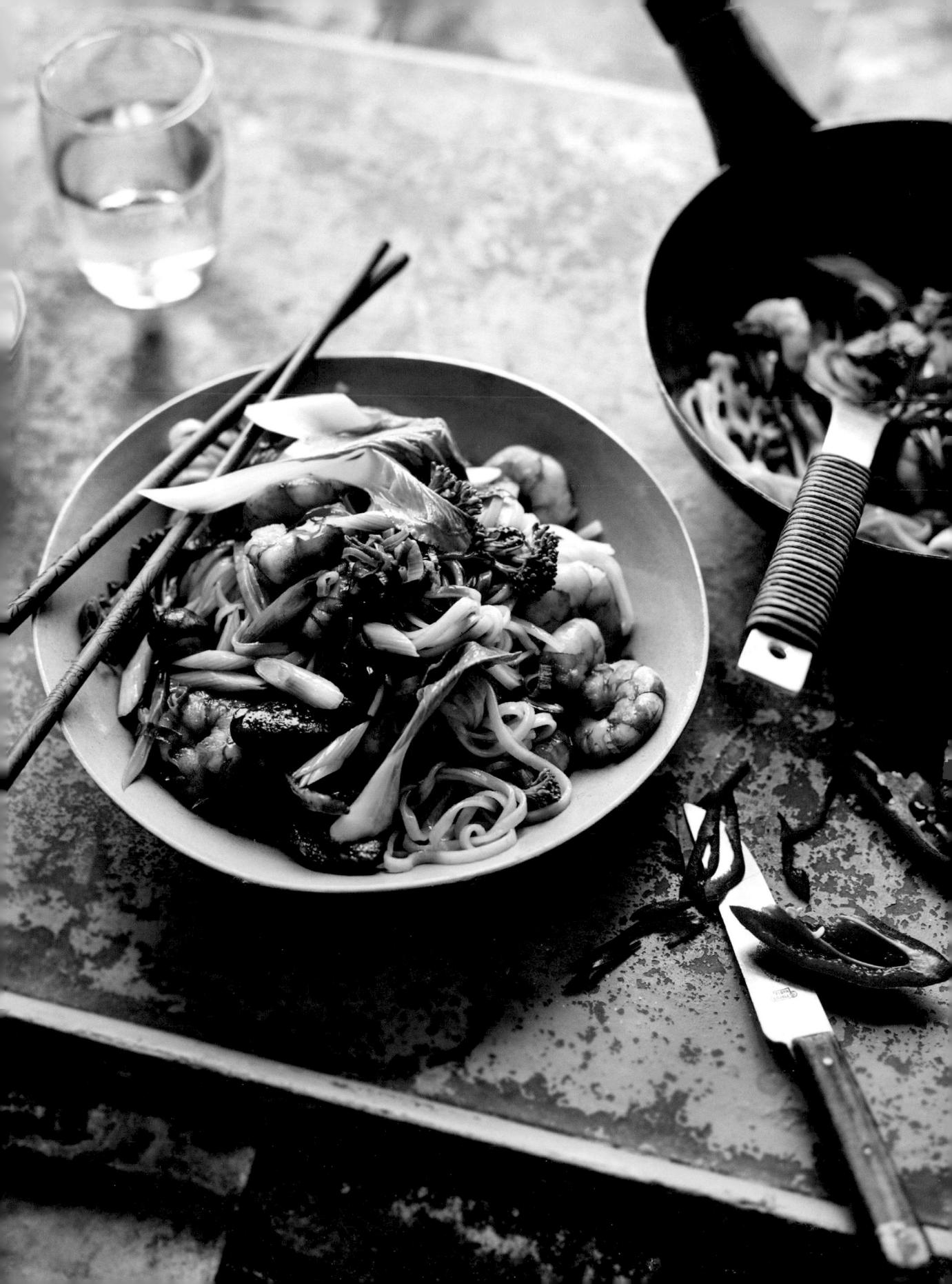

Lamb Tikka Flatbreads with Herb Salad

This is a recipe that I think everyone will love. It's got it all going on. Invite some friends over and cook it for them, too!

Ingredients

2 tbsp tikka curry paste
juice of ½ lemon
½ tsp grated ginger
250g lean lamb leg steaks (all visible fat removed)
salt and pepper
1 large naan bread or large Middle Eastern flatbread, warmed
1½ tbsp zero-fat Greek-style yoghurt, whisked with 1 tsp lemon juice (optional)

For the herb salad

¼ cucumber, de-seeded and cut into 1cm dice
1 plum tomato, cut into 1cm dice
¼ red onion, finely diced
3 tbsp mint, finely chopped, plus extra for garnish
3 tbsp coriander, finely chopped, plus extra for garnish
juice of ½ lemon
1 green chilli, de-seeded and finely chopped

Method

Place the tikka curry paste, lemon juice and ginger in a wide glass bowl.

Cut the lamb into small bite-sized cubes and toss them in the tikka paste mixture. Season.

Meanwhile, make the herb salad by mixing together all the ingredients in a bowl. Season and set aside.

Preheat the grill to medium-high.

Thread the marinated lamb onto one or two metal skewers and place them under the grill. Cook for 8–10 minutes, turning once halfway through, until cooked and lightly charred at the edges.

Remove the lamb from the skewers with a fork and scatter onto the warmed naan or flatbread.

Spoon over the herb salad and drizzle over the yoghurt mixture (if using). Sprinkle with the chopped mint and coriander before tucking in.

Post-workout

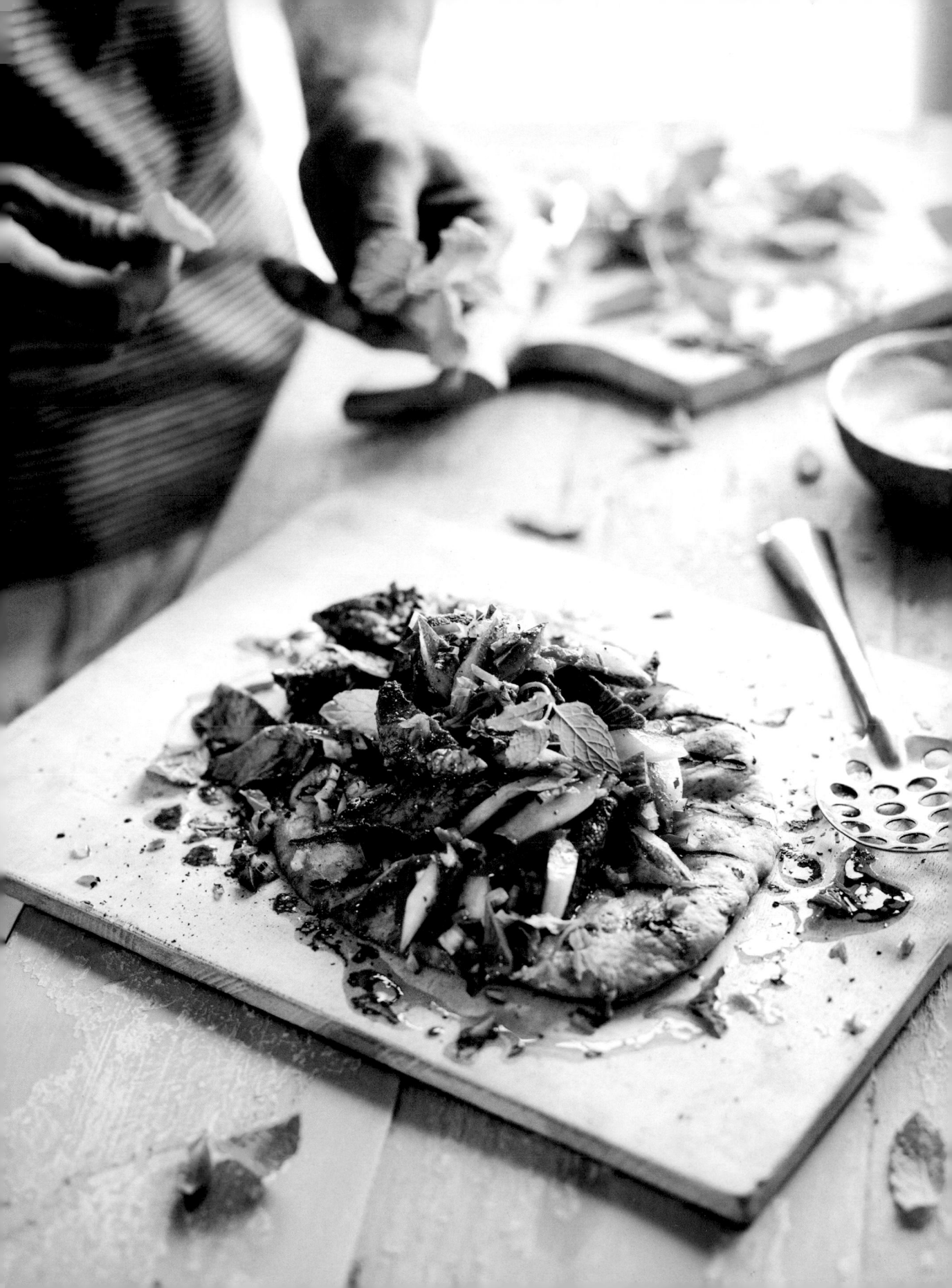

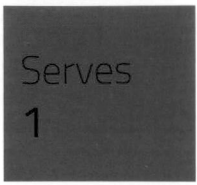 Make ahead

Ingredients

95g penne pasta
½ tbsp coconut oil
225g extra-lean beef
 steak mince
¼ carrot, very finely diced
 or grated
1 celery stick, very finely diced
2 cloves garlic, crushed
8–10 baby button mushrooms,
 thinly sliced or halved or
 quartered
2 tbsp sundried tomato puree
½ x 400g tin of chopped
 tomatoes
1 tsp golden caster sugar
100ml boiling hot beef stock
1 tsp dried Italian herb
 seasoning
¼ tsp dried red chilli flakes
salt and pepper
small handful basil leaves,
 roughly torn, for garnish

Quick Bolognese with Penne

A simple classic which never lets you down. The bolognese will keep in the fridge for 2 days in a sealed container, so feel free to double the recipe to prep like a boss.

Method

Cook the penne according to packet instructions.

Melt the oil in a large non-stick frying pan over a high heat. Brown the mince for 1–2 minutes, then throw in the carrot, celery, garlic and mushrooms and soften for 3 minutes.

Stir in the sundried tomato puree, tomatoes, sugar, stock, dried herbs and chilli flakes. Season well and bring to the boil, then simmer for 10 minutes until thickened and reduced.

Drain the cooked pasta and place in a bowl. Serve with the sauce and torn basil leaves scattered on top.

Post-workout

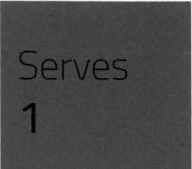

Serves
1

Griddled Chicken with Truffle Mash

Truffle is a love-it-or-hate-it flavour for many people. I personally love the stuff but feel free to leave it out from the mashed potato if you prefer. The recipe will still taste awesome without it.

Ingredients

150g potatoes, peeled and cut
  into small pieces
1 x 180g skinless
  chicken breast fillet
salt and pepper
½ tbsp coconut oil, melted
½ tsp truffle oil
small handful of wild
  rocket leaves
4 tbsp tinned cannellini beans,
  rinsed and drained

For the salsa verde

1 tsp finely grated lemon zest
  and juice of 1 lemon
3 tbsp basil, finely chopped
3 tbsp flat-leaf parsley,
  finely chopped
½ tbsp tarragon,
  finely chopped
½ tbsp capers, rinsed
  and drained
½ clove garlic, crushed
2 tsp Dijon mustard

Method

Cook the potatoes in a pan of boiling water for 10–12 minutes, or until tender. Drain the potatoes, return to the pan and mash until fairly smooth.

Place the chicken between two pieces of cling film, and using a rolling pin or wooden mallet, lightly beat until about 1cm thick. Season well and lightly brush all over with the coconut oil.

Cook on a preheated non-stick griddle pan for 4–5 minutes on each side, or until cooked through and lightly charred at the edges.

Meanwhile, make the salsa verde by whizzing all the ingredients in a food processor. Season and set aside.

Stir the truffle oil into the warm mash and spread the mash on a plate, topped with the rocket and beans. Slice the chicken and place it on top.

Drizzle over the salsa verde and serve.

Post-workout

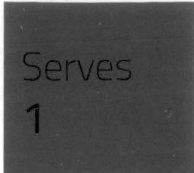

Toasted Ciabatta with Fillet Steak and Harissa

Sometimes after a workout you just want to get in and out of the kitchen as quickly as possible. This recipe will do just that, and when you walk away with this ciabatta in your hands, you'll feel like a winner.

Ingredients

250g lean beef steak
1 tbsp rose harissa paste
salt and pepper
100g (drained weight) tinned borlotti beans, rinsed and drained
2 tbsp vegetable stock
1 tbsp parsley, finely chopped
2 individual ciabatta buns
2 tbsp onion marmalade
1 plum tomato, sliced
small handful of wild rocket

Method

Place the steak between two pieces of cling film, and using a rolling pin or wooden mallet, lightly beat until about 1cm thick. Remove the cling film, put the meat in a bowl and rub with the harissa and a pinch of sea salt.

Chuck the beans in a small food processor with the stock and parsley and blend until it makes a thick and fairly smooth spreadable paste.

Heat a griddle pan over a medium to high heat. Halve the ciabatta buns, and griddle on both sides until golden and charred. Set aside.

Leave the pan over a medium to high heat and sear the steak for 1–2 minutes on each side for rare, or 3 minutes on each side for medium–well done. Remove and rest the meat for 5 minutes.

To serve, spread the bean and herb paste onto the base of each bun, and top with the onion marmalade. Place the tomato slices on top.

Thinly slice the steak. Divide it between the buns and top with the rocket and the ciabatta buns.

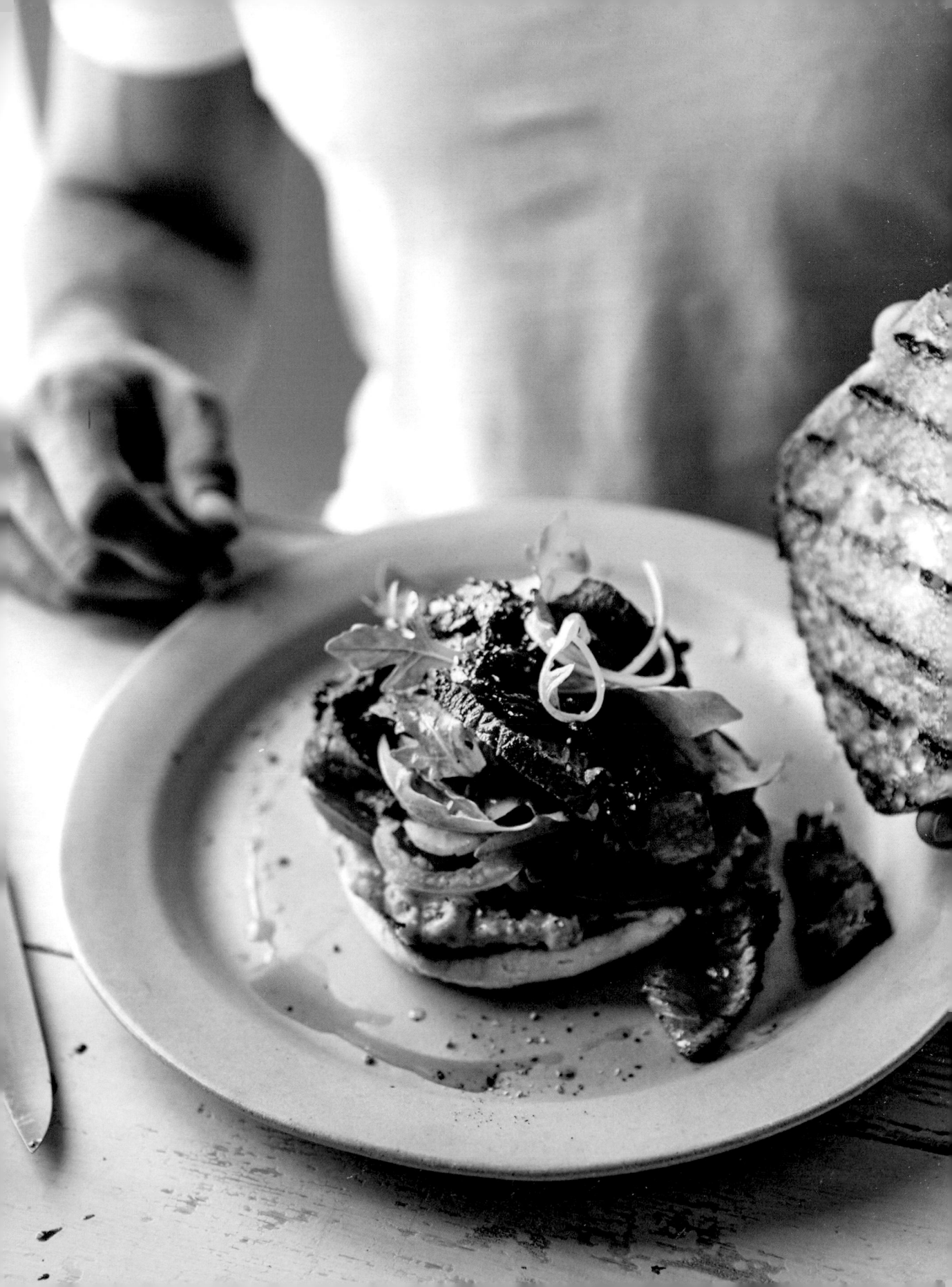

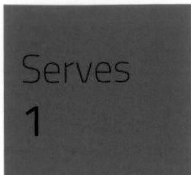
Mexican Cod Tacos with Pineapple Salsa

If you haven't tried fish tacos before, you should give this recipe a go. They taste so fresh and make use of so many lovely spices and flavours.

Ingredients

1 x 250g skinless cod
  loin fillet
salt and pepper
½ tbsp coconut oil
2 corn tortillas
small handful of watercress

For the spice rub

1 tsp sweet smoked paprika
½ tsp garlic powder
½ tsp ground cumin
½ tsp dried oregano
1 tbsp plain flour

For the salsa

100g fresh pineapple,
  cut into 1cm dice
½ small red onion, very
  finely diced
1 red chilli, de-seeded and
  finely diced
2 tbsp coriander, finely
  chopped
juice of 1–2 limes

Method

Put the cod fillet onto a plate and season with salt. Slice the fish into 3cm pieces and put into a bowl.

Mix all the spice rub ingredients together in a small bowl, then toss in the cod, turning the pieces to evenly coat in the rub.

Chuck all the salsa ingredients into a bowl, season well and set aside.

Melt the oil in a large non-stick frying pan. Add the fish and fry for 2–3 minutes. Turn the fish carefully, trying not to break it up too much (it will need 4–5 minutes in total), then remove and set aside.

Rub the pan with kitchen roll. Add the tortillas and fry for a minute on each side to warm or cook the tortillas over a very hot non-stick, ridged griddle pan until lightly griddle-marked and warmed through.

To serve, divide the watercress between the warmed tortillas, top with the fish and spoon over the salsa. Roll up and tuck in.

Post-workout

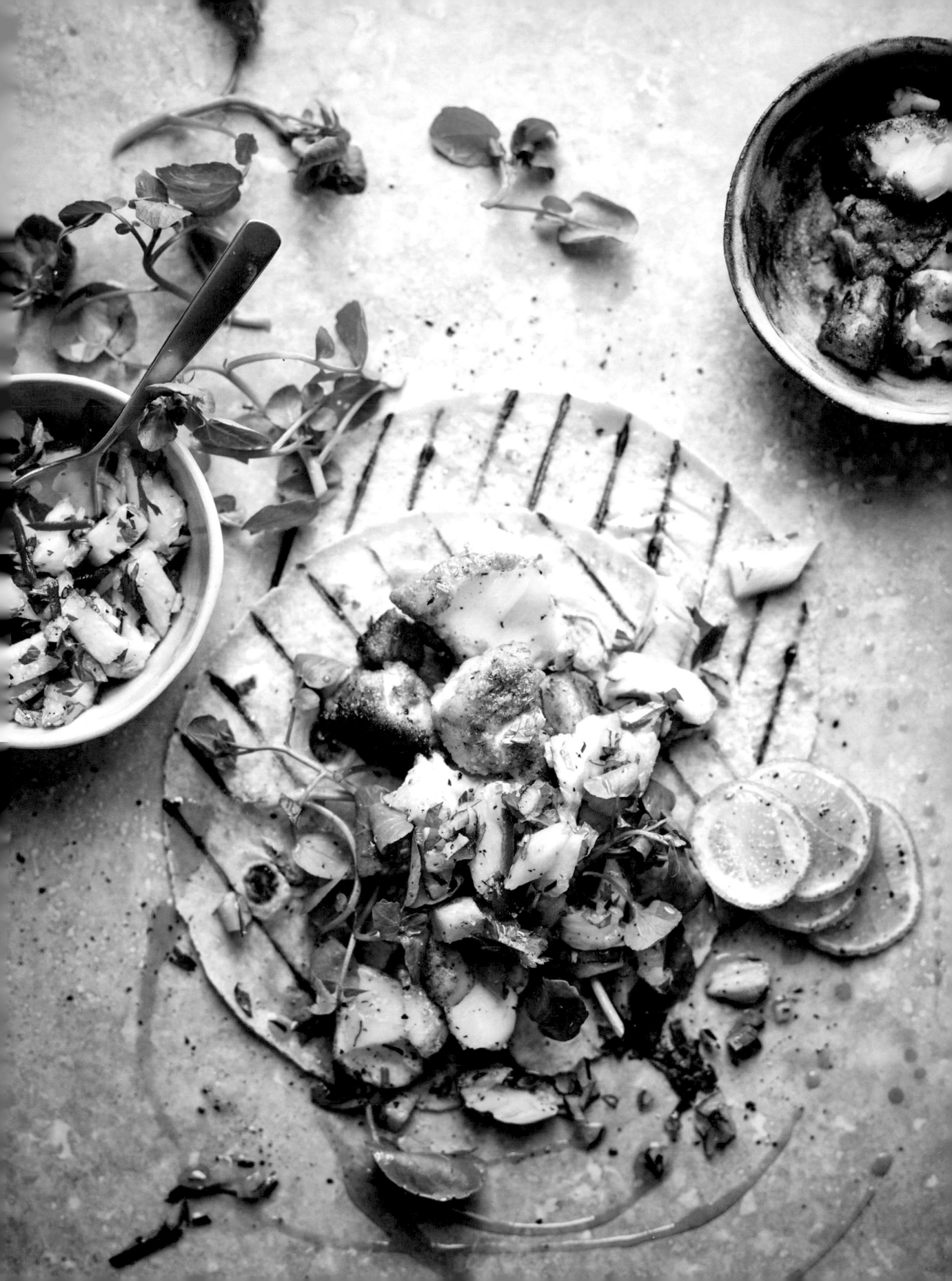

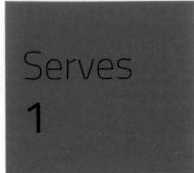

Steak with Caramelised Onions and Sweet Potato Fries

This recipe speaks for itself. It looks unreal and tastes even better. Just what you want to smash after a workout.

Ingredients

1 sweet potato, peeled and cut into thin chips
1 tbsp coconut oil
2 tbsp rich beef stock
2 tbsp dark soy sauce
1 tbsp Dijon mustard
1 tsp dark muscovado sugar
250g lean minute or sandwich steak, cut into strips
salt and pepper
1 onion, thinly sliced
1 tbsp balsamic vinegar
1 thick slice of good-quality sourdough bread
1 clove garlic, peeled and halved
small handful of lamb's lettuce, to serve

Method

To make the sweet potato fries, preheat the oven to 200°C (fan 180°C/gas mark 6). Line a baking tray with baking parchment.

Place the sweet potato fries on the tray and toss with ½ tablespoon of the coconut oil. Spread the fries out evenly and bake for 12–15 minutes until tender.

Meanwhile, mix the stock, soy sauce, mustard and sugar in a big bowl. Toss in the steak strips, season well with pepper and leave to sit and marinate while you get everything else ready.

Melt the remaining oil in a large non-stick frying pan over a medium heat. Add the onion and balsamic, turn up the heat to very high and cook for 3–4 minutes, stirring frequently until lightly caramelised. Transfer the onions to a plate and keep them warm.

Lift the steak strips out of the marinade with a slotted spoon and stir-fry them in the onion pan over a very high heat for 1 minute (do it in two batches if it's easier).

Pour in the marinade from the bowl and boil for a few seconds until it sticks to the meat but is still juicy. Season with salt and pepper and keep warm.

Toast the bread and then rub the halved clove garlic over it. Cut the bread in half and place it on your plate.

Top with a spoonful of onions, then the steak and more onions. Put a little pile of lamb's lettuce on each plate and serve with sweet potato fries.

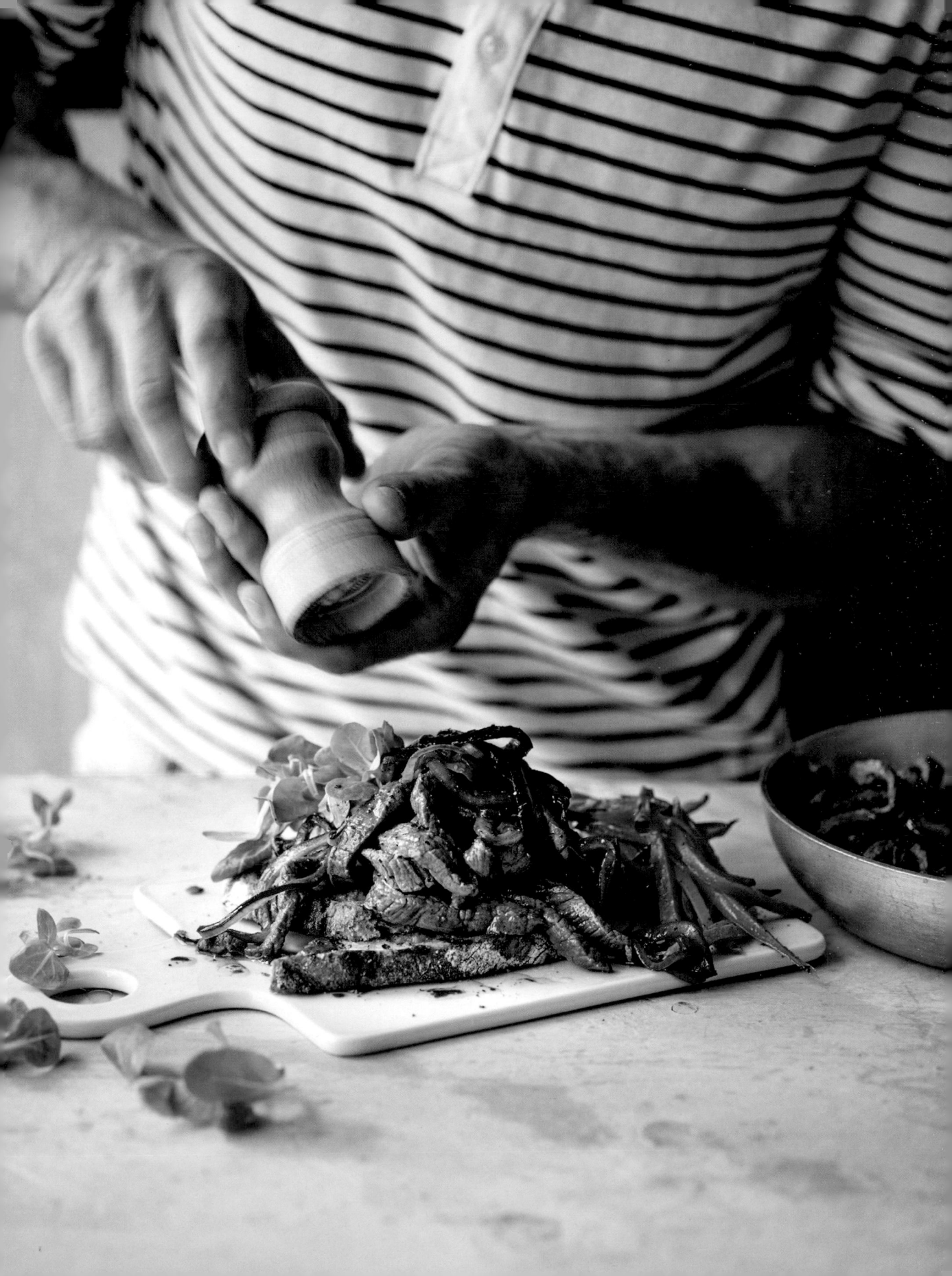

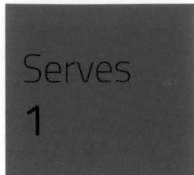

Serves
1

Beef, Shiitake and Spring Onion Risotto

A risotto usually takes a long time but by using pre-cooked rice I've made this recipe much quicker. With coriander, chilli and soy sauce there's plenty of flavour.

Ingredients

½ tbsp coconut oil

225g extra-lean beef
  steak mince

5 shiitake mushrooms, sliced

½ red pepper, de-seeded and
  finely diced

2 cloves garlic, crushed

1 tsp finely grated ginger

4 spring onions, finely sliced

100ml boiling hot beef or
  chicken stock

250g pre-cooked basmati rice

2 tbsp light soy sauce

1 tsp sesame oil

large handful of coriander,
  finely chopped

salt and pepper

1 tsp finely diced red chilli,
  for garnish

Method

Melt the oil in a wide non-stick frying pan over a high heat. Add the beef and stir and cook for 4–5 minutes, or until browned.

Add the mushrooms, red pepper, garlic, ginger and spring onions and stir and cook for 3–4 minutes or until the mushrooms are tender.

Stir in the stock and rice and stir and cook for 3–4 minutes, or until piping hot.

Stir in the soy sauce and sesame oil, remove from the heat and stir in the coriander.

Season and serve topped with the red chilli.

Post-workout

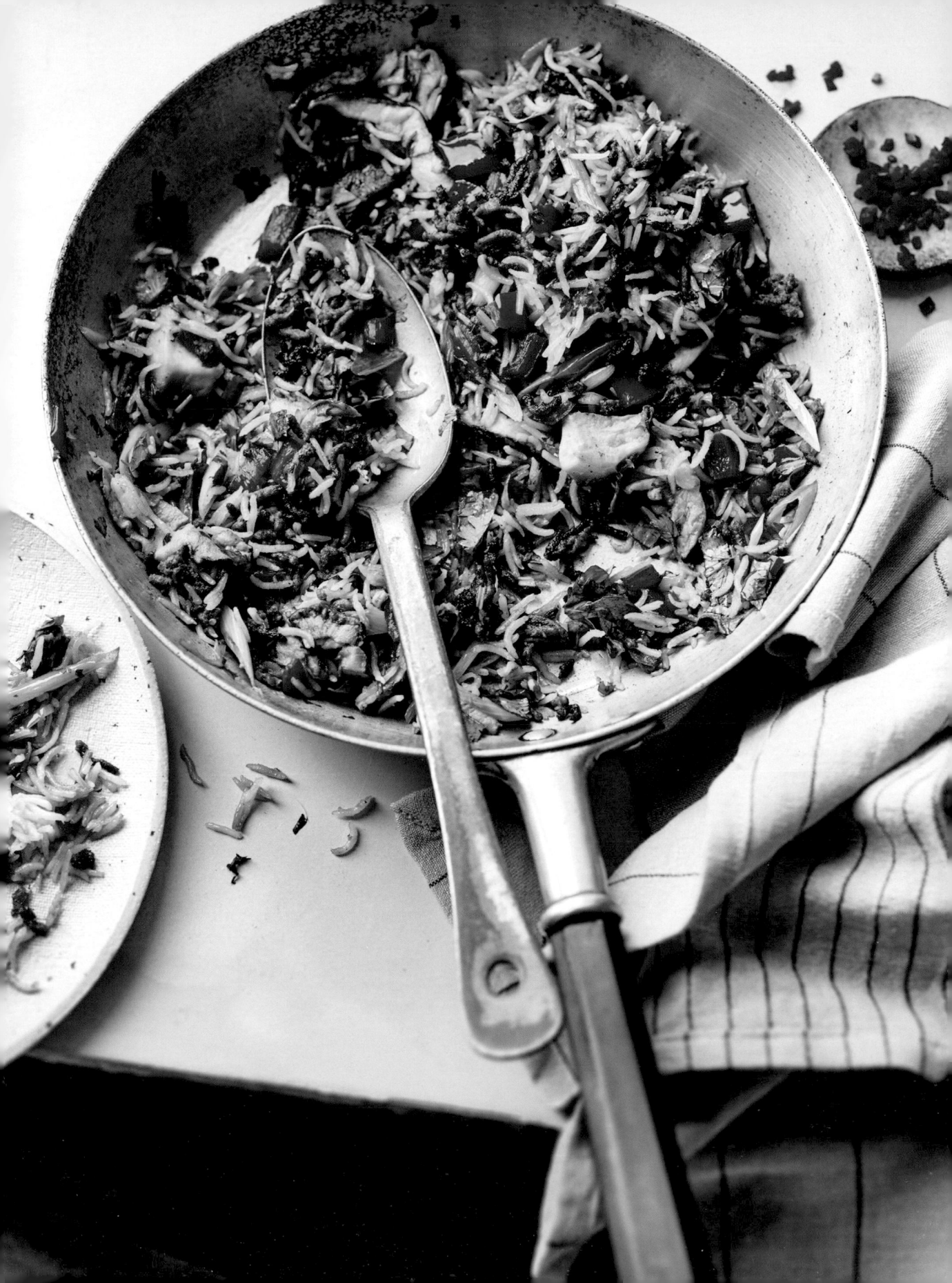

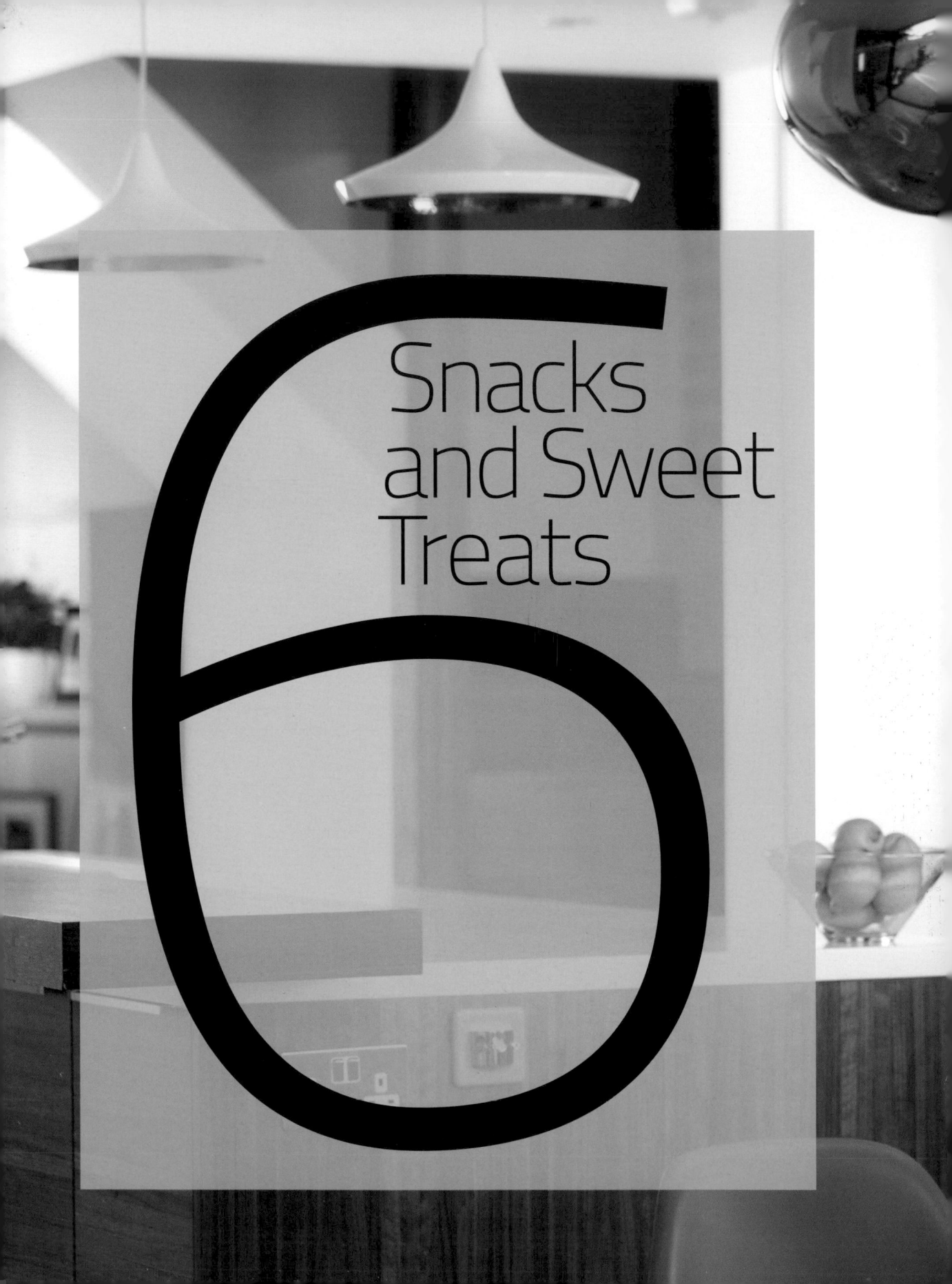

6 Snacks and Sweet Treats

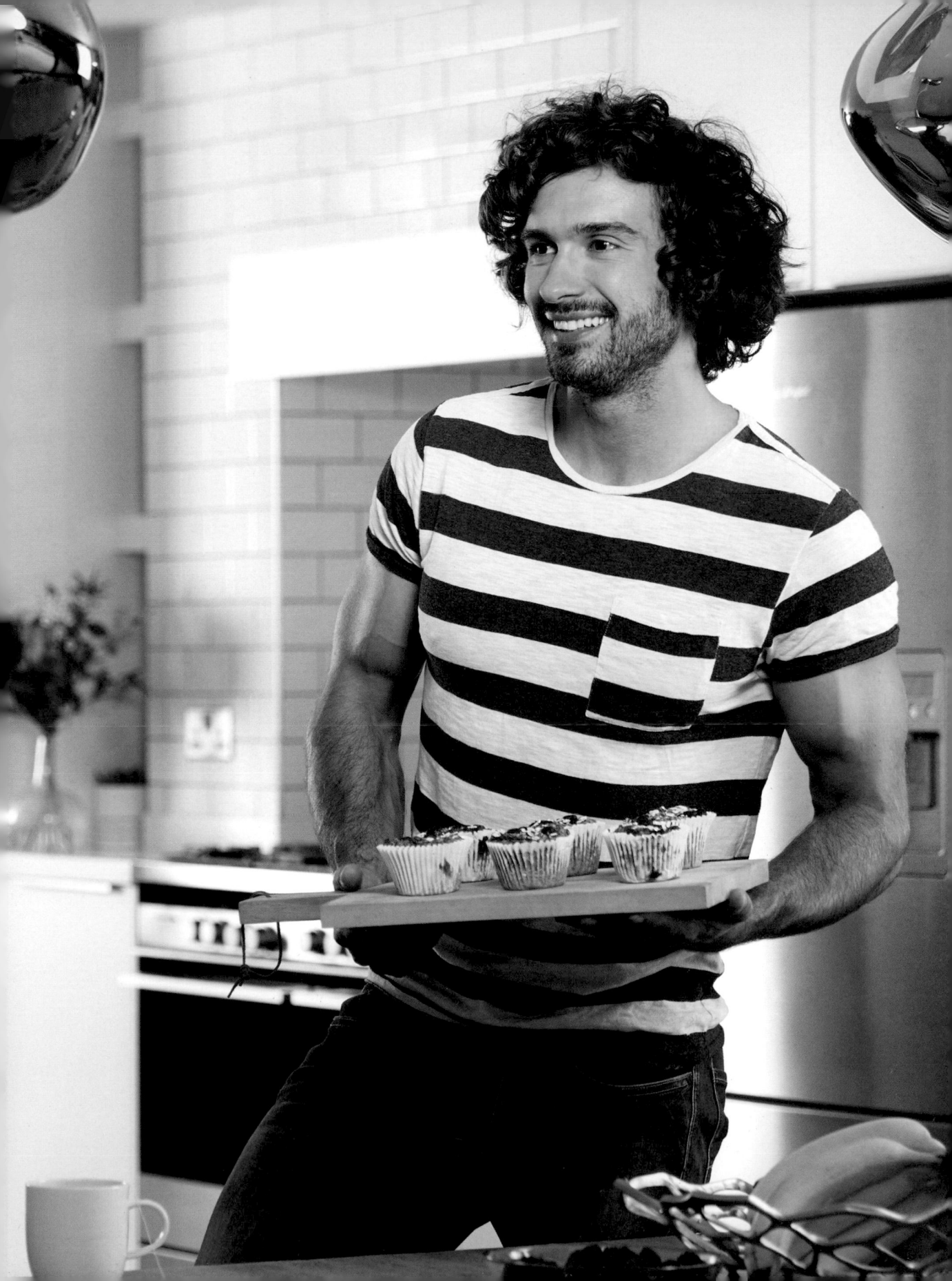

Avocado Hummus with Super Seed Dukkah

This is a really tasty snack with plenty of healthy fats to provide you with energy for the day.

Ingredients

finely grated zest and
  juice of 1 lemon
1 tbsp tahini paste
2 cloves garlic, crushed
1 x 400g tin of chickpeas,
  drained
1 ripe avocado, de-stoned
  and chopped
1 tbsp mint leaves,
  finely chopped
1 tbsp coriander leaves,
  finely chopped
1 tbsp extra-virgin olive oil,
  to drizzle
vegetable sticks and warm
  strips of pitta bread, to serve

For the super seed dukkah

2 tsp cumin seeds
2 tsp sesame seeds
1 tsp fennel seeds
2 tbsp blanched almonds,
  chopped

Method

Preheat the oven to 180°C (fan 160°C/gas mark 4).

To make the dukkah, place the seeds and nuts in a roasting tin and roast for 4–5 minutes. Allow to cool. Lightly crush with a rolling pin and set aside.

Place the lemon zest and juice in a small food processor with the tahini, garlic, chickpeas, avocado and chopped herbs. Pulse until well combined but still slightly chunky.

Spoon into a shallow bowl and scatter over the dukkah. Top with a drizzle of the olive oil and serve with the vegetable sticks and pitta bread. The hummus will keep for 2 days in an airtight container in a fridge.

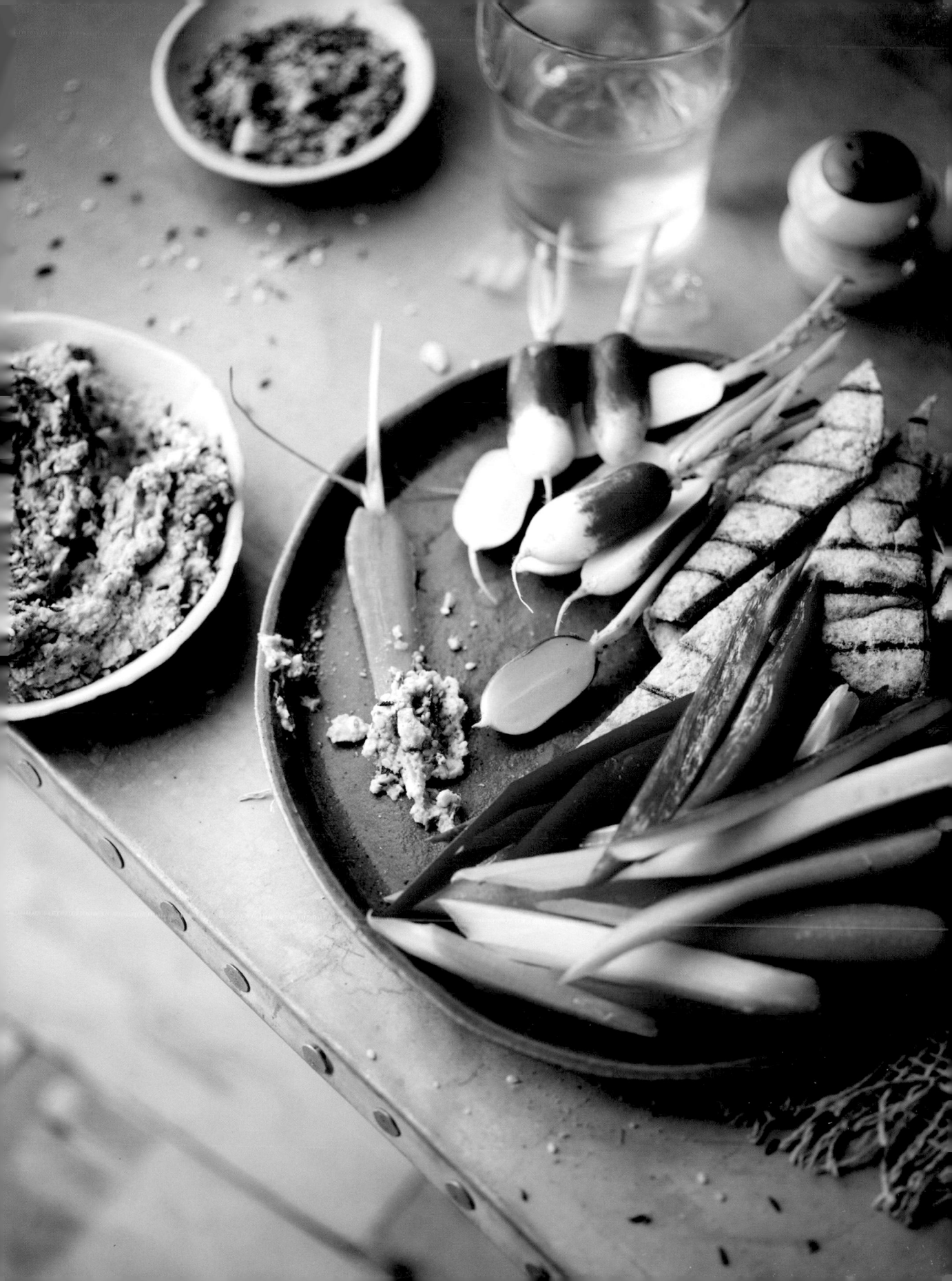

Coconut and Almond Macaroons

Beware, these are very moreish. In fact, during the recipe testing, I accidentally ate all eighteen. Guilty, Your Honour.

Ingredients

2 medium egg whites
50g coconut sugar
115g desiccated coconut
115g ground almonds
1 tbsp vanilla protein powder
**30g white chocolate, broken
  into pieces**

Method

Line two baking trays with baking parchment, and preheat the oven to 170°C (fan 150°C/gas mark 3).

In a very clean bowl, whip the egg whites until they form soft peaks. Gently fold through the coconut sugar using a metal spoon.

Add the coconut, almonds and protein powder and combine until you have a sticky dough.

Spoon out eighteen even-sized dollops across the two baking trays and bake for 15 minutes until golden brown. Remove from the oven and leave to cool on a wire rack.

Melt the chocolate in a glass bowl over a pan of boiling water, making sure the bowl doesn't touch the water. Using a teaspoon, quickly drizzle over the cooked macaroons. Store in an airtight container.

Tip For a dairy-free alternative, use a vegan protein powder and top each one with an almond before baking. Omit the white chocolate.

Oaty Blueberry Muffins

If you're craving a sweet treat, give this recipe a go. They are so easy to make and taste awesome. If you've got young kids they also make a good breakfast for them.

Ingredients

100g jumbo oats, plus 1 tablespoon to decorate
40g ground almonds
10g chia seeds
1 tsp baking powder
¼ tsp bicarbonate of soda
pinch of salt
4 medjool dates, de-stoned and torn into pieces
1 small ripe banana
150ml almond milk
1 tsp vanilla extract
100g blueberries

Method

Preheat the oven to 180°C (fan 160°C/gas mark 4) and line a 6-hole muffin tin with paper cases.

In a food processor, pulse the oats until they are a similar consistency to flour.

Tip the oats into a large mixing bowl and stir through the ground almonds, chia seeds, baking powder, bicarbonate of soda and salt.

In the same food processor (you don't need to wash it after the oats), blend the dates until they form a thick paste. Add the banana and pulse until mashed, then pour in the milk and vanilla extract. Pulse a few times until mixed together.

Pour the wet mixture into the dry ingredients, scraping down the sides of the food processor. Add 75g of the blueberries and fold it all together until just combined.

Divide the mixture between the muffin cases and scatter with the leftover blueberries and oats. Bake in the middle of the oven for 20 minutes, or until an inserted skewer comes out clean. Allow to cool on a wire rack, then serve.

Make ahead

Joe's Little Balls of Energy

One or two of these are great little treat, but try not to eat too many in one sitting as they do contain loads of energy. Even healthy treats can put you in a calorie surplus and stop you burning fat.

Ingredients

2 tbsp coconut oil
1 tbsp maple syrup
2 tbsp cashew butter
¼ tsp ground cinnamon
100g cashew nuts
50g desiccated coconut
100g medjool dates, de-stoned
  and chopped

Method

Melt the coconut oil in a saucepan, then remove from the heat. Stir in the maple syrup, cashew butter and cinnamon until smooth.

Grind the cashews in a mini food processor until fairly finely chopped (some should turn into powder, but you still want a few chunks). Transfer to a bowl and stir in half the coconut.

Add the dates to a small food processor then add the cashew butter mixture and blend to a paste. Stir this into the nut mixture in the bowl.

Scatter the rest of the coconut on a large plate. Taking 1 tablespoon of the date paste at a time, roll into sixteen balls. Roll in the desiccated coconut to coat and chill, covered, for about 1 hour, or until firm.

Store in an airtight container.

Tip These freeze really well! Place in a single layer in a zip-lock bag, on a tray in the freezer. This will stop them clumping together. After an hour you can remove the tray and store them more compactly. Allow to defrost for about 20–25 minutes before eating.

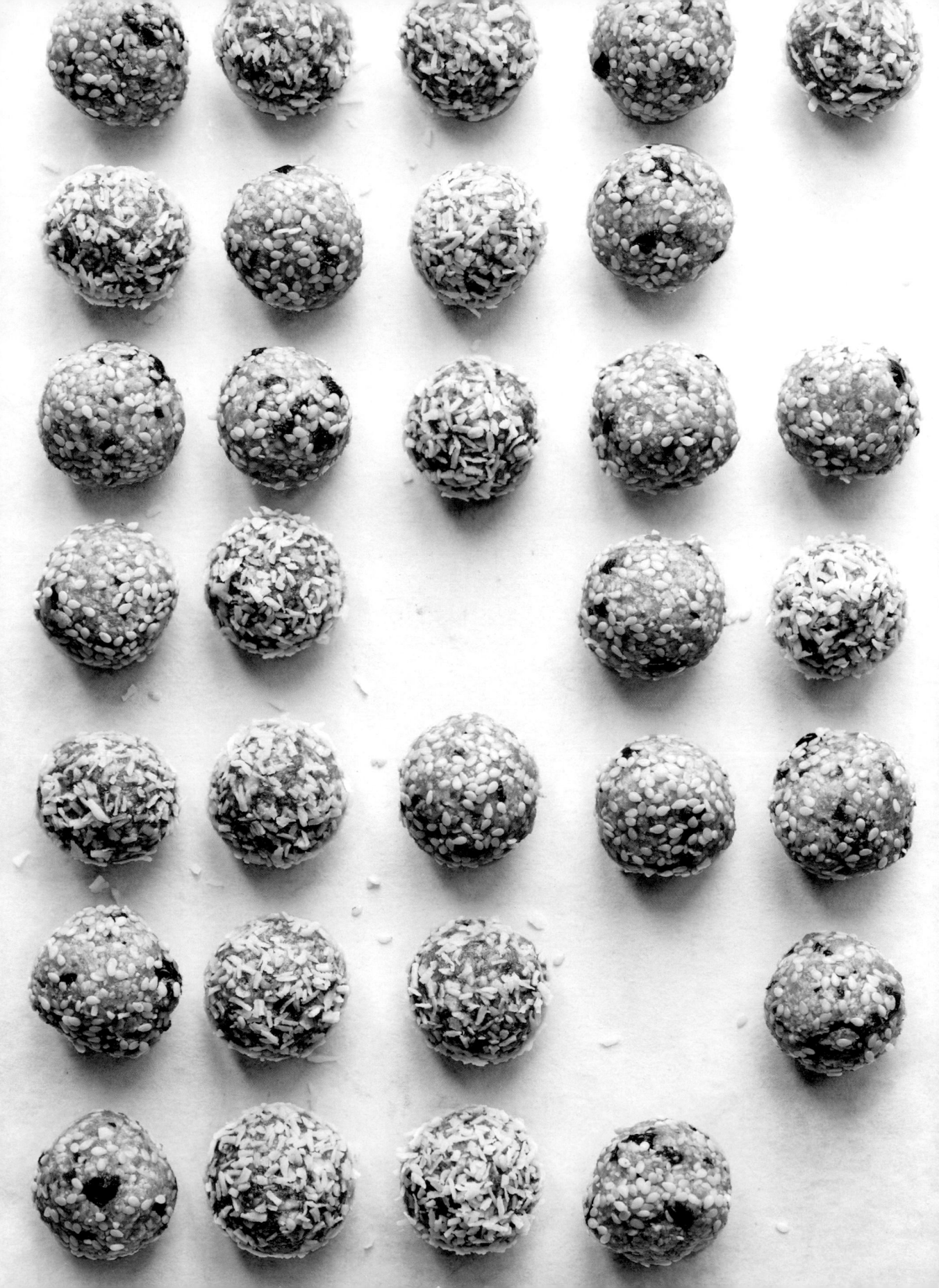

🕐 Make ahead

Ingredients

150g cashew nuts
20g desiccated coconut
140g dried apricots
1 tbsp vanilla protein powder
35g dried cranberries
20g sesame seeds (optional)

Cashew and Coconut Energy Balls

Here's another version of the ever-popular energy balls. They are very energy dense so one or two per serving is ideal.

Method

Pulse the cashews in a blender until they are finely chopped. Add the coconut, apricots and protein powder and blend for about a minute, until you reach a chunky consistency that sticks together when squeezed.

Add the cranberries and pulse a few times until they are slightly chopped and mixed evenly through the mixture.

Roll into sixteen even-sized balls, coating in sesame seeds if you wish (you will have to press these into the balls after you roll them in the seeds to get them to stick).

Store in an airtight container. See freezing instructions on page 192.

Pineapple and Coconut Ice Cream Lollies

These taste good all year round, so go on, give them a try and treat yourself.

Ingredients

200g ripe pineapple flesh
1 tbsp sweetened condensed milk
100ml pineapple juice
1 tbsp icing sugar (optional)
150ml coconut milk

Method

Chop the pineapple flesh into 1cm dice and divide between eight 100ml ice lolly moulds.

Pour the condensed milk, pineapple juice, icing sugar (if using) and coconut milk into a food processor and blend until smooth. Transfer to a measuring jug and carefully pour into the ice lolly moulds to come up to 1cm from the top of the moulds.

Cover the tops of the moulds with tin foil and make a small slit in the centre of the foil on each mould. Carefully insert the lolly sticks into the moulds through the prepared slits.

Freeze for 8 hours or overnight until set. To unmould, briefly dip the moulds in warm water for 10–15 seconds and serve.

Enjoy the ice lollies immediately or store them in airtight sealable freezer bags in the freezer. You can also keep them frozen in their moulds for up to 1 week.

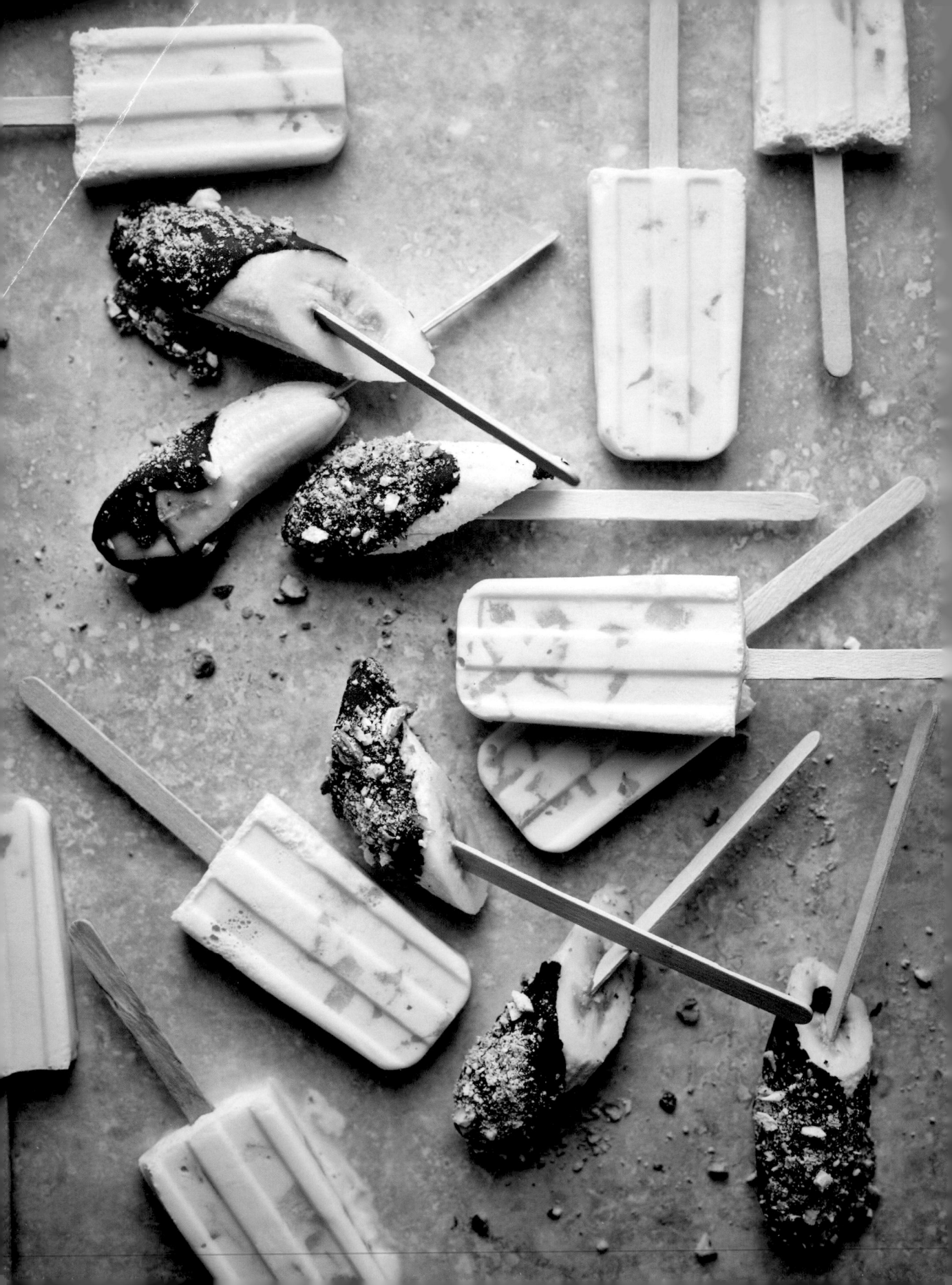

Choco-nut Banana Popsicles

These are so fun to make and they taste awesome. The kids will enjoy making these with you. I use pistachio nuts here but you could use chopped cashews, macadamias or walnuts.

Ingredients

100g dark chocolate, broken into small pieces
3 large bananas
60g pistachio nuts, finely chopped

Method

Melt the dark chocolate in a heatproof bowl over a saucepan of barely simmering water.

Cut each banana into four chunks on the diagonal. Push a wooden lolly stick into the end of each one. Dip each banana piece into the melted chocolate so they are half covered and transfer them to a baking sheet lined with baking parchment. Sprinkle with the chopped pistachios.

Freeze for 1 hour, or until solid. Take out of the freezer 10–15 minutes before eating. Keep them for up to 2 weeks in the freezer.

OMG Chocolate Orange Popcorn Squares

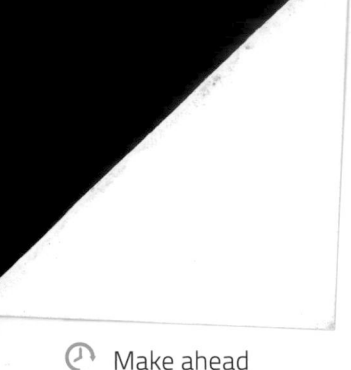

🕐 Make ahead
🖤 Naughtee

This is my favourite sweet treat in the whole book. They are a bit of a naughtee treat so be sure to enjoy them now and again and not every day if you want to get lean.

Ingredients

¼ tsp coconut oil
3 tbsp popping corn
150g dark chocolate, broken into small pieces
75g butter, cubed
75g golden syrup
4 tsp finely grated orange zest
40g white chocolate

Method

Line an 18cm square, loose-bottomed cake tin with non-stick baking parchment.

In a large non-stick lidded saucepan, melt the oil over a medium heat. Add the popping corn.

Cover and cook, shaking the pan frequently until the corn has popped.

Place the dark chocolate, butter and golden syrup in a glass bowl set over a pan of gently simmering water (making sure that the water does not touch the base of the bowl). Allow to melt and stir to combine.

When the chocolate is smooth, stir in half of the orange zest.

Mix the popcorn with the chocolate mixture to coat evenly and then spoon the mixture into the prepared tin, pressing down firmly with the back of a spoon. Chill for 1–2 hours, or until set.

Carefully turn out the mixture onto a board and remove the paper. Melt the white chocolate as above and drizzle all over. Sprinkle over the remaining zest. Then transfer to the fridge and chill until the white chocolate has set.

Using a sharp knife, cut into sixteen equal squares and serve.

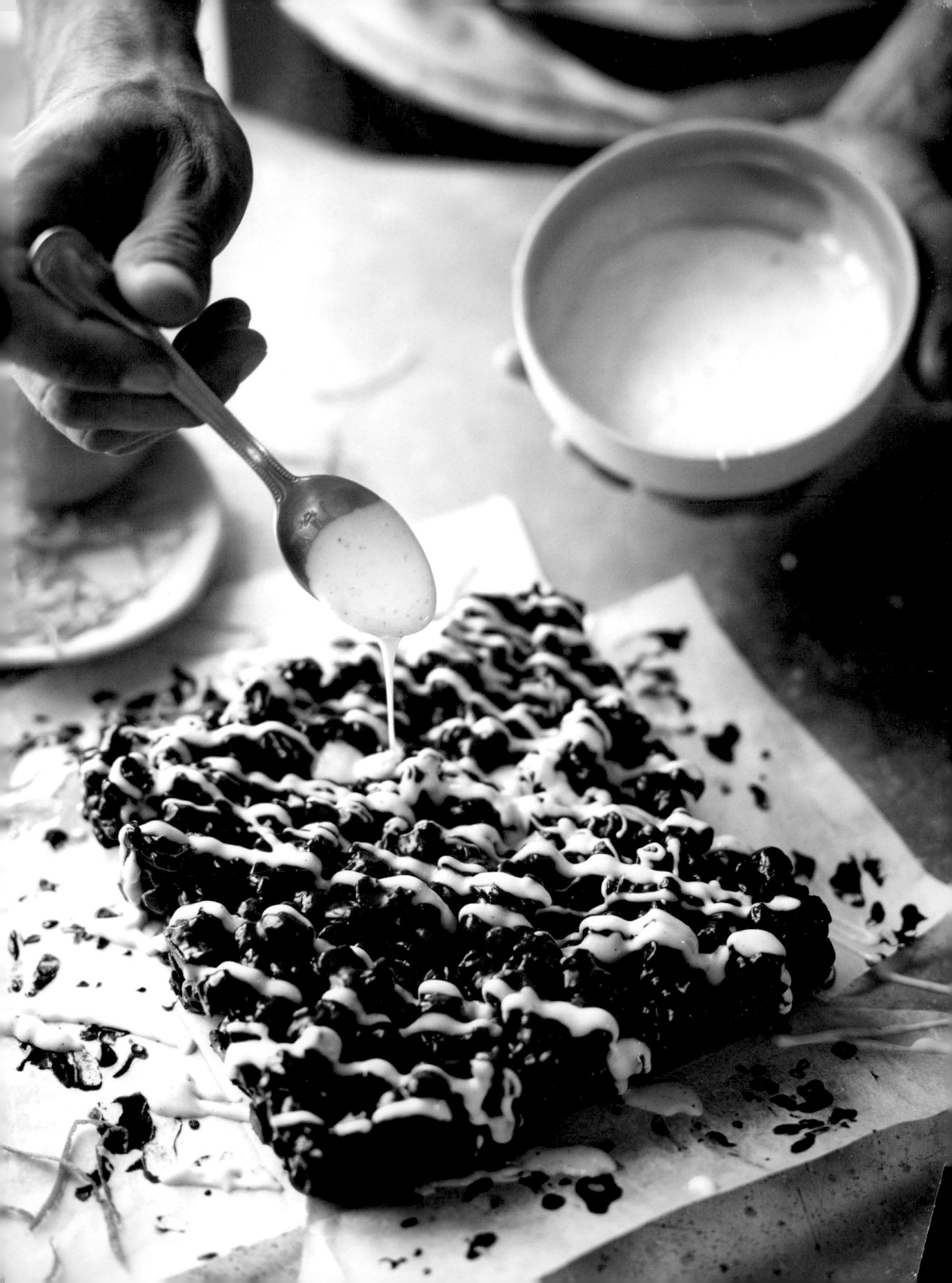

**Makes
12**

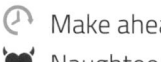 Make ahead
Naughtee

Ingredients

100g unsalted butter
50g coconut sugar
1 medium egg
1 tsp vanilla extract
150g plain flour
50g white spelt flour
1 tsp baking powder
pinch of salt
100g milk chocolate chips

Joe's Naughtee Choc-chip Cookies

These taste delicious, but beware, they are extremely addictive. Luckily you bake the cookies from frozen, so you can be sensible and only make a small batch when you need a little treat.

Method

Start by making the brown butter. In a pan with a light-coloured bottom (so you can see as the colour changes), melt the butter over a medium heat. Swirl the butter around the pan occasionally to help the butter to cook uniformly.

As the butter starts to brown, it will foam. Skim to one side so you can keep an eye as the butter turns from yellow to brown. When the butter is a dark tan colour and has started to smell nutty, remove the pan from the heat and pour into a bowl to cool. Try to leave as many of the dark dregs (the cooked milk solids) in the pan as possible, as these can be discarded.

Line two baking trays with baking parchment. When the butter has cooled, mix in the coconut sugar, egg and vanilla extract.

In a second bowl, mix together the flours, baking powder, salt and chocolate chips. Pour the wet ingredients into this bowl and mix with a wooden spoon until combined.

Roll the mixture into twelve even-sized balls, and flatten each one out. Place them on the baking trays.

Freeze the cookies for 30 minutes to an hour. Preheat the oven to 160°C (fan 140°C/gas mark 3). Once they are frozen, you can either cook them straightaway on the trays or store in a zip-lock bag in the freezer until you want them.

Bake from frozen for 15 minutes, until golden brown on the outside and still slightly soft inside. Allow to cool on a wire rack, then store in an airtight container for up to 1 week.

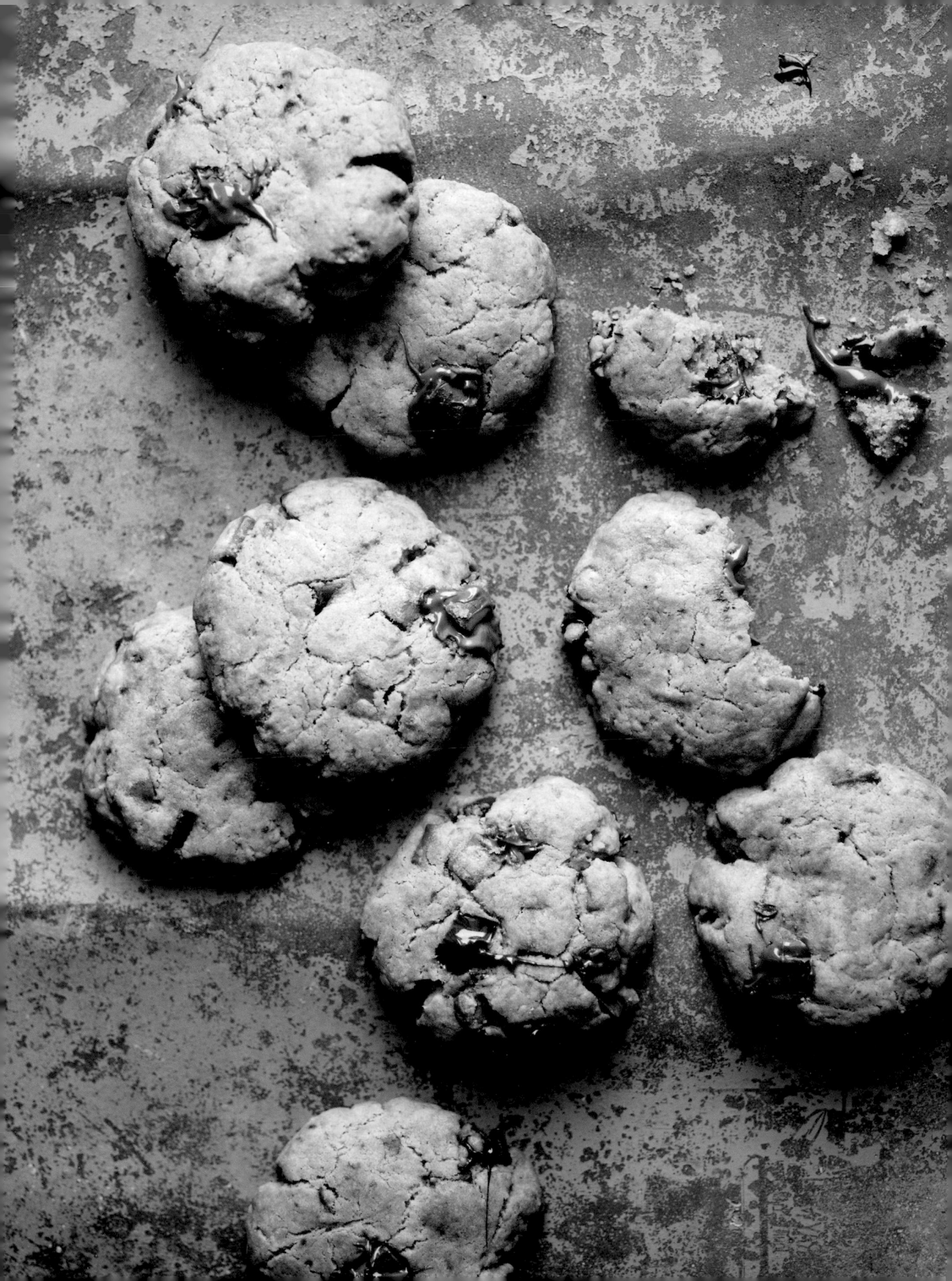

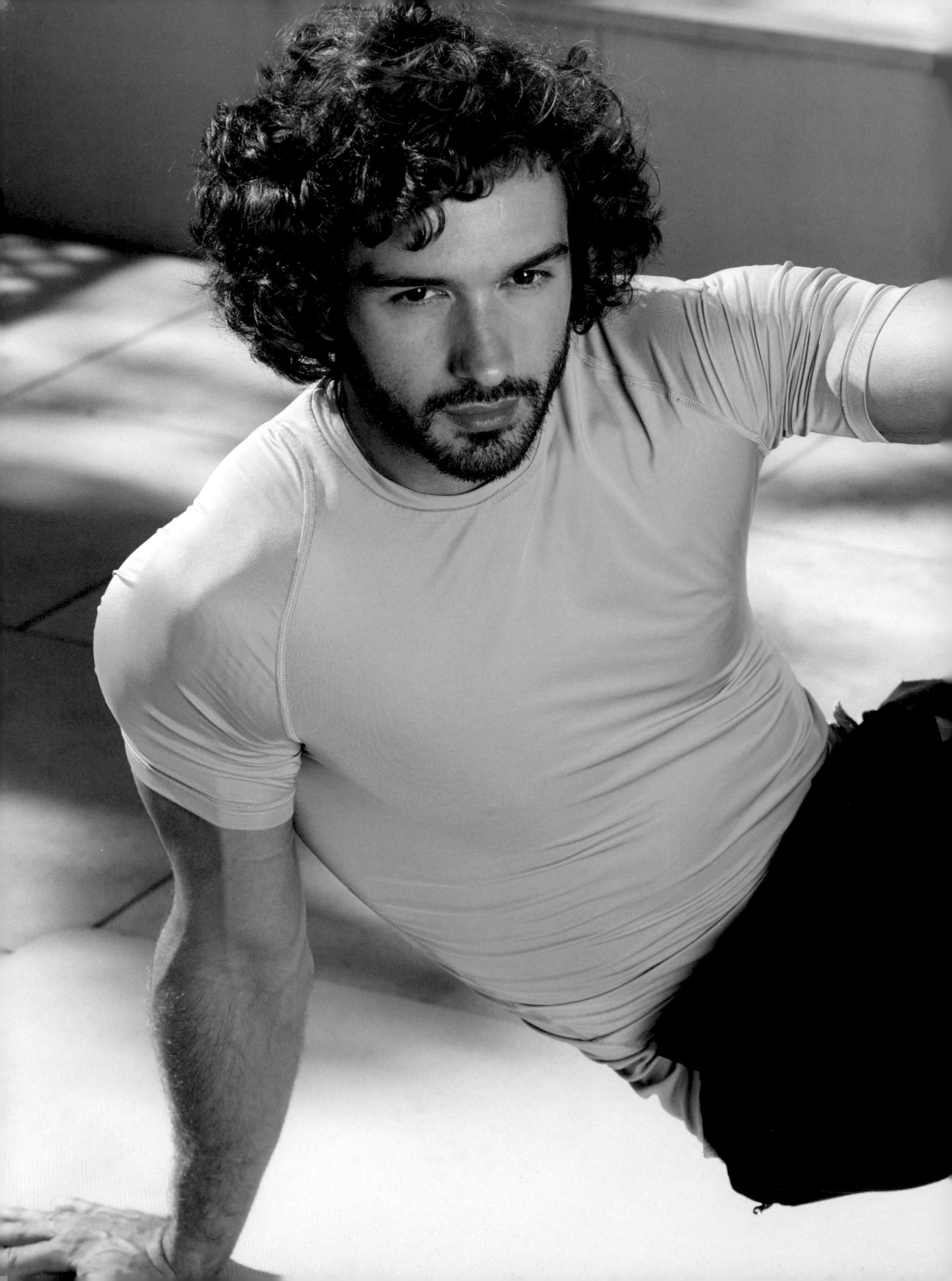

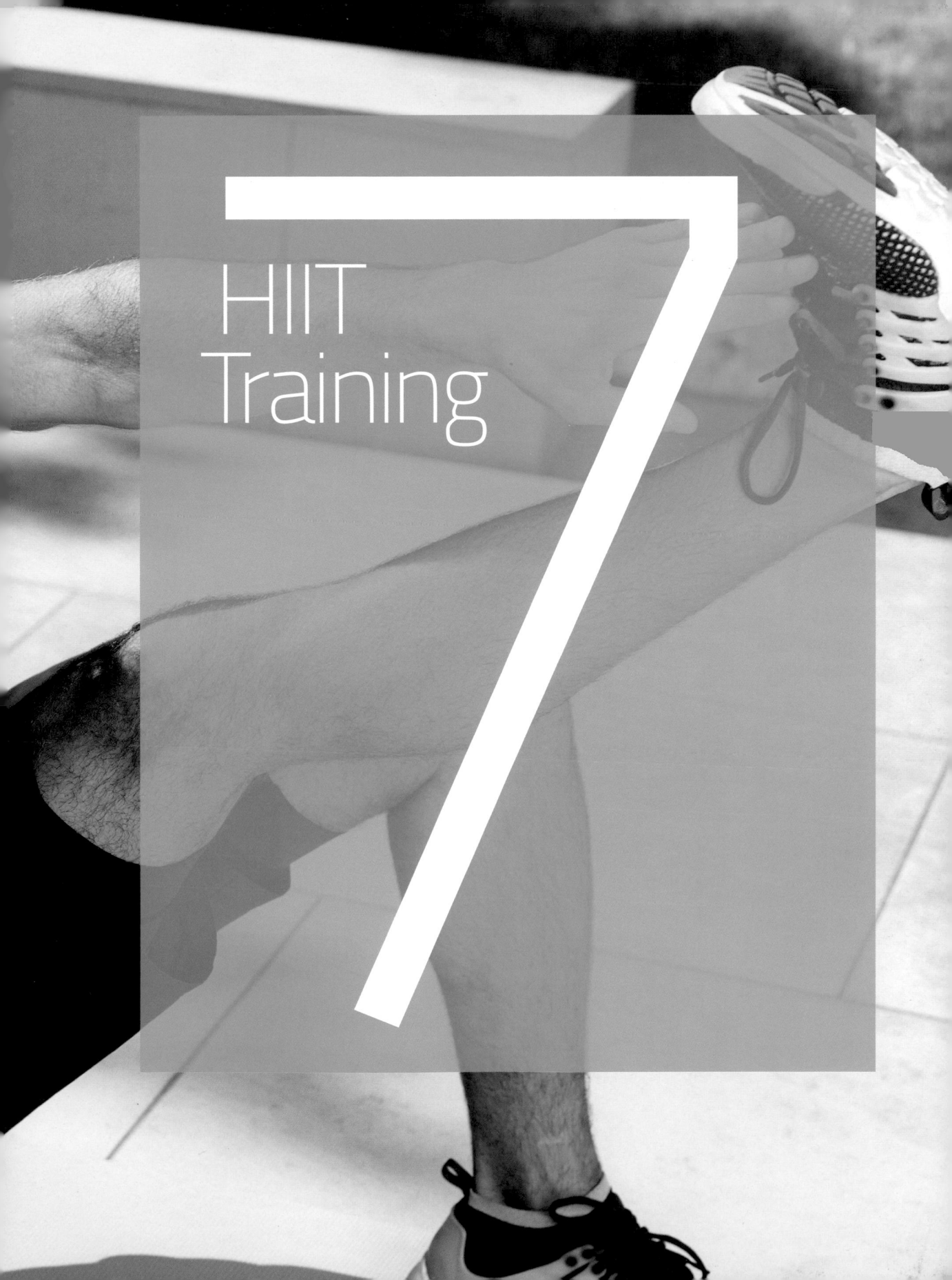

HIIT
Training

7

The Fat-Loss Training Plan

For the best results this training plan involves five sessions per week and two full rest days. But please don't shy away if you don't feel you could really fit that into your life right now. It's not a problem. Even if you can only manage three workouts per week you can still get your body burning fat. It will just take you a bit longer to reach your goal, that's all.

There's no expiry date or end point to this – it's the never-ending plan and just continues all year round. This is going to become a part of your lifestyle now and you'll be feeling fit and confident all year round instead of panicking two weeks before your summer holiday and doing some awful crash diet.

How to train

The training plan combines both HIIT cardio with resistance training. This is because I believe that in order to have a fit, strong and healthy body a combination of both is ideal.

You'll notice I have listed the work:rest ratios for beginner, intermediate and advanced levels of fitness. This allows you to gauge your current levels of fitness by having a longer rest period to begin with. Then as you get fitter you can try doing more rounds and with less rest between exercises. This will really step up the intensity of a HIIT and get you super fit.

Example week

Aim to perform three HIIT sessions and two weight sessions per week in any order. You can choose from the HIIT bodyweight workouts one and two, or any HIIT machine workout. Perform weight-training workout one and weight-training workout two each week.

Beginners will workout for 18 minutes, intermediate for 24 minutes, advanced for 30 minutes.

Monday	**HIIT machine cardio**
Tuesday	Weight-training workout 1
Wednesday	**Bodyweight HIIT workout 1**
Thursday	REST DAY
Friday	**Weight-training workout 2**
Saturday	Bodyweight HIIT workout 2
Sunday	**REST DAY**

1. Climb the rope

Start by running on the spot. Lift your knees as high as possible then imagine you are reaching up above your head to pull a rope down towards your body. Do this as fast as possible.

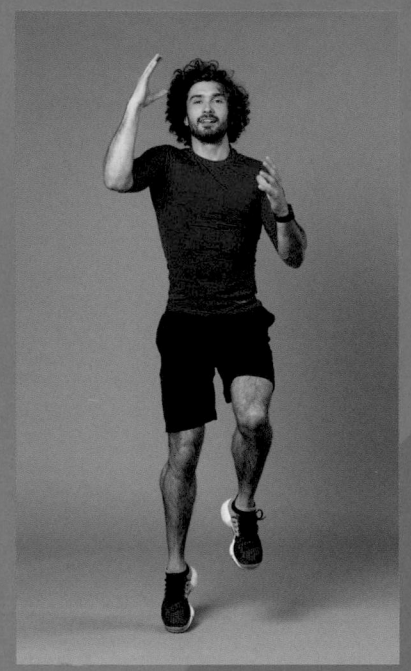
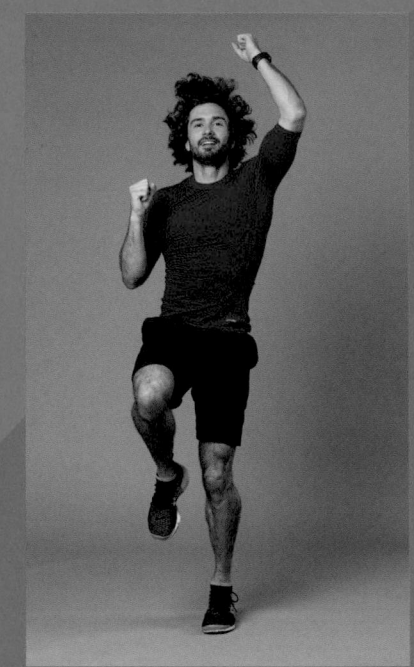

2. Squat thrusts

Start in a strong plank position with your core engaged and back straight. Then jump both feet forward towards your hands. Kick them back out again into the plank and repeat as fast as possible.

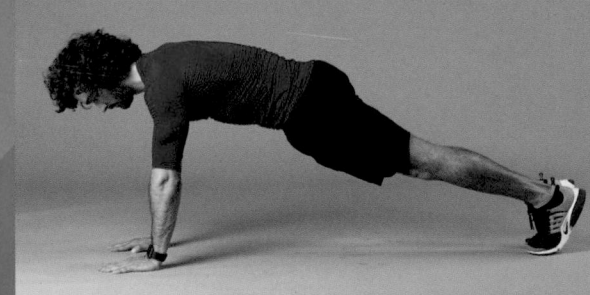
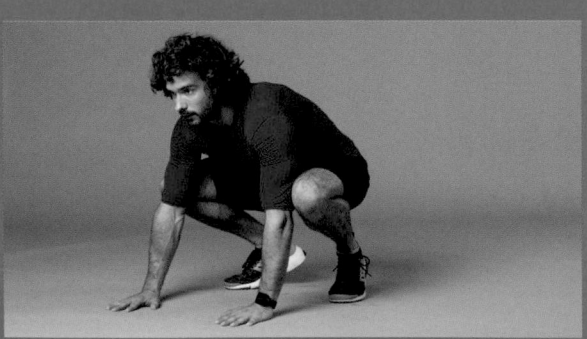

3. Power squats

This one is a real leg-burner. Drop down fast, taking your feet wide into a low squat and then drive up, bringing your feet together and arms above your head. Repeat.

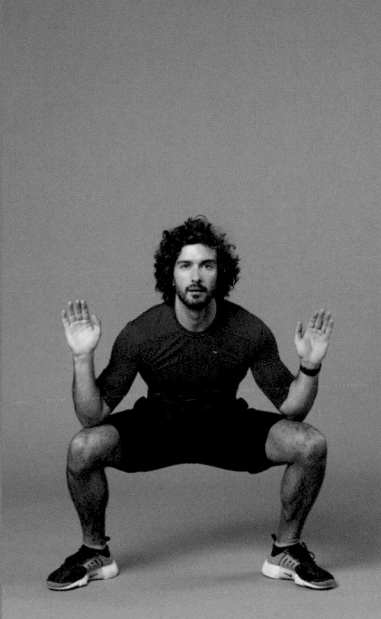
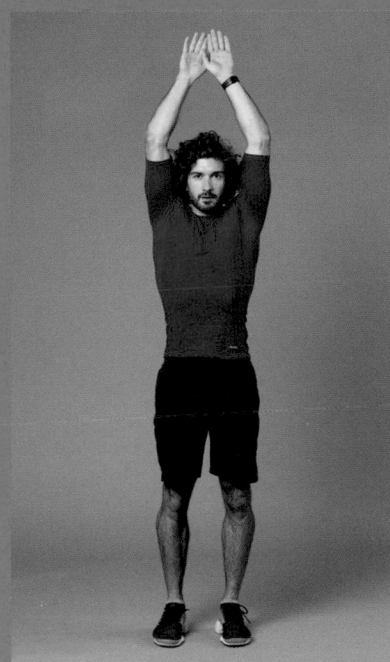

4. Press ups

Keep your abs engaged to prevent your lower back arching as you lower your chest to the ground and push up to straighten your arms.

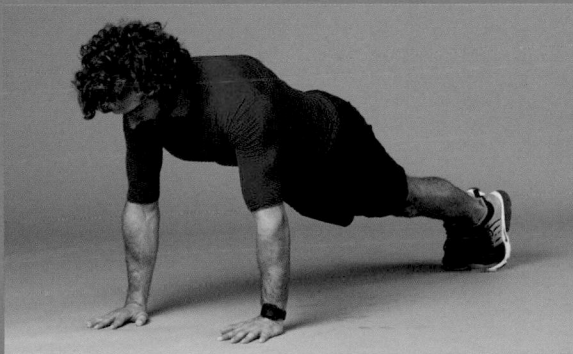
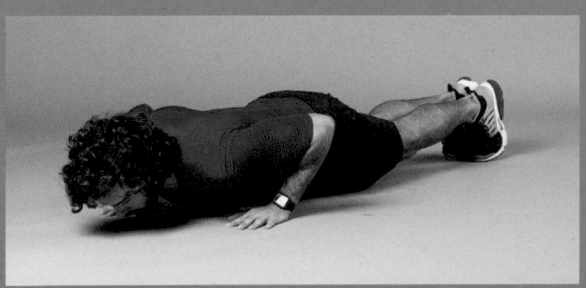

4. Burpees

Love it or hate it, the burpee
is one of the best full-body
cardio moves to get your heart
pumping and your body burning
fat. They never feel easy but are
worth the effort.

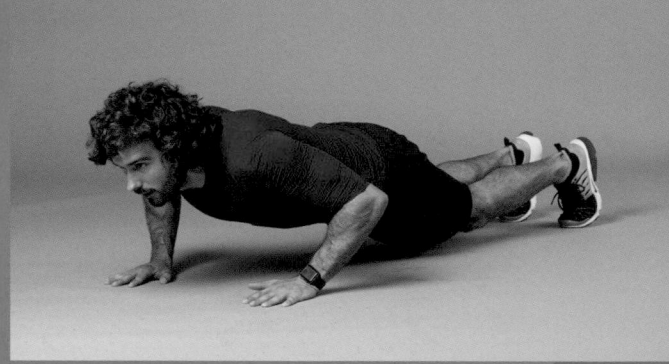

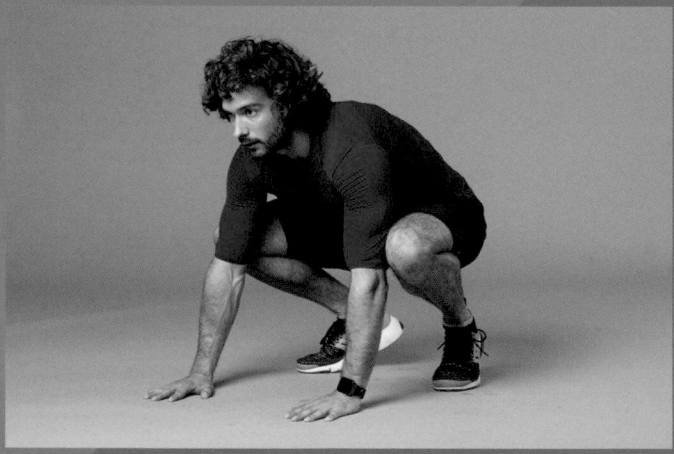

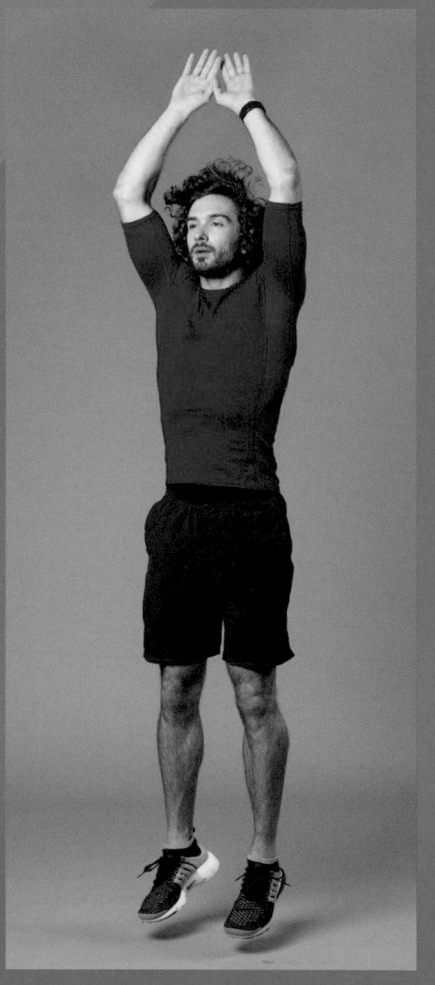

5. Toe touches

Aim to lift your body off the ground and keep your bum off the floor and alternate between kicking your foot up to touch your toes. Left hand meets right foot and vice versa.

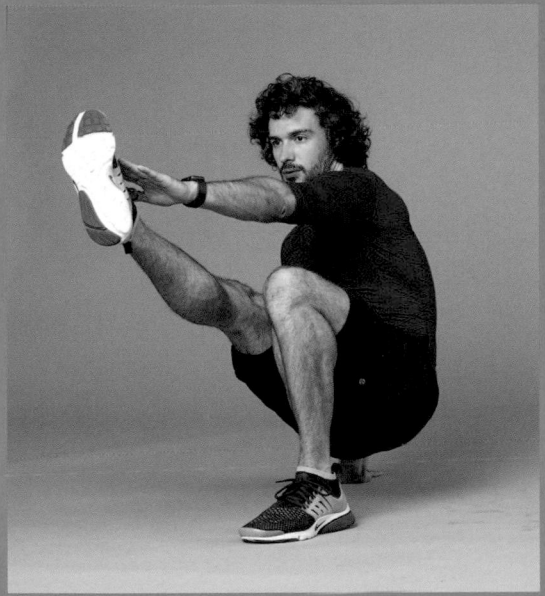 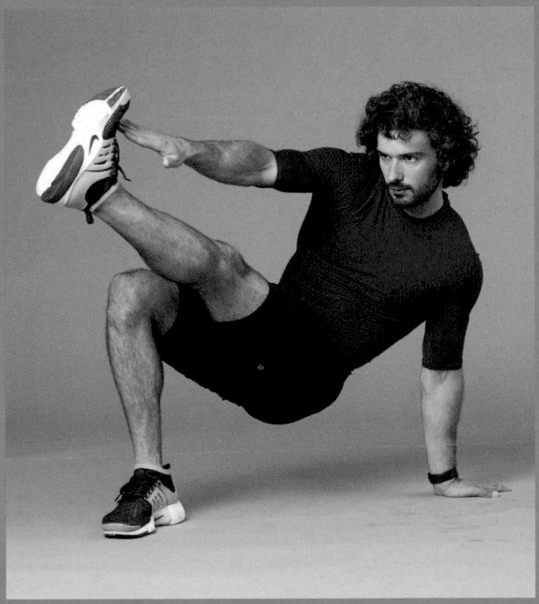

Beginner (3 rounds)	Intermediate (4 rounds)	Advanced (5 rounds)
20 seconds work	30 seconds work	40 seconds work
40 seconds rest	30 seconds rest	20 seconds rest

Bodyweight HIIT Workout 2

1. Mountain climbers

Be sure to keep your abs engaged to prevent your back from dipping and arching. Avoid sticking your bum up in the air. Keep a flat back and, one at a time, drive your knees towards your chest as fast as you can.

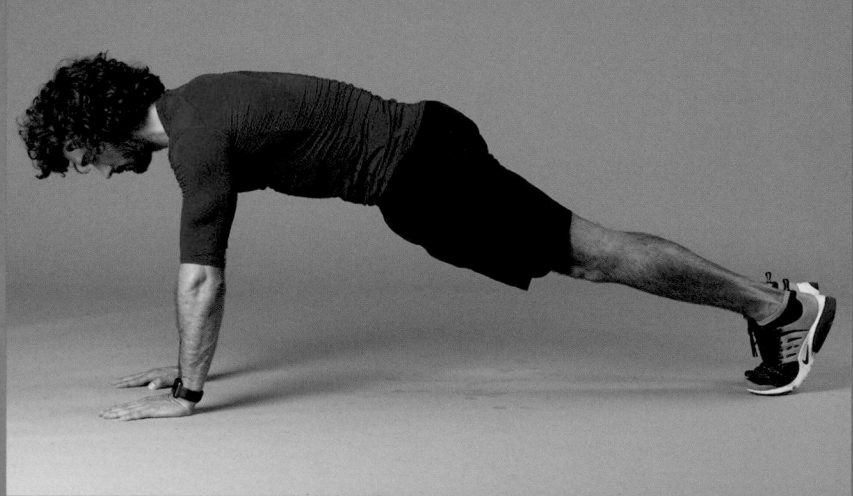

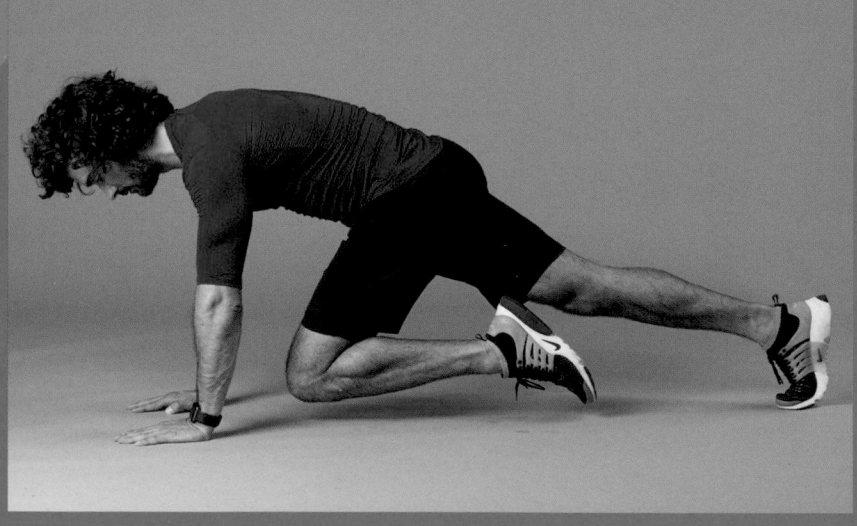

2. Lateral shuffle floor touches

Simply shuffle left and right as quick as you can and touch the floor each time. Focus on bending the legs to get your legs working, as opposed to just bending forward from the hips.

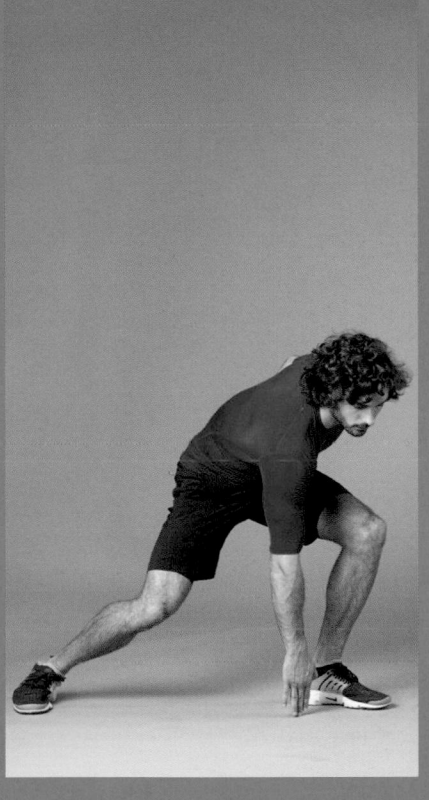
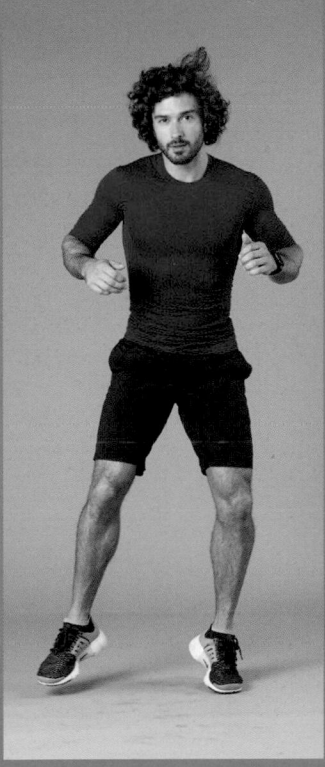
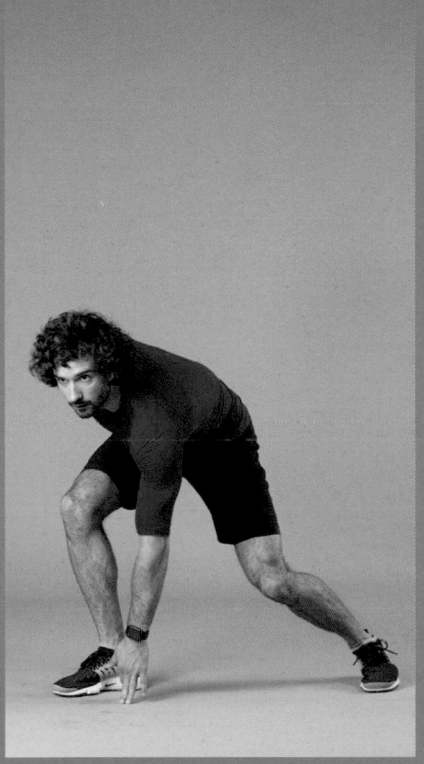

3. Single leg hops

Step back into a reverse lunge,
lowering your knee towards
the ground. When your hand
touches the floor you then
drive up with the front leg into
an explosive hop. Alternate
between both legs.

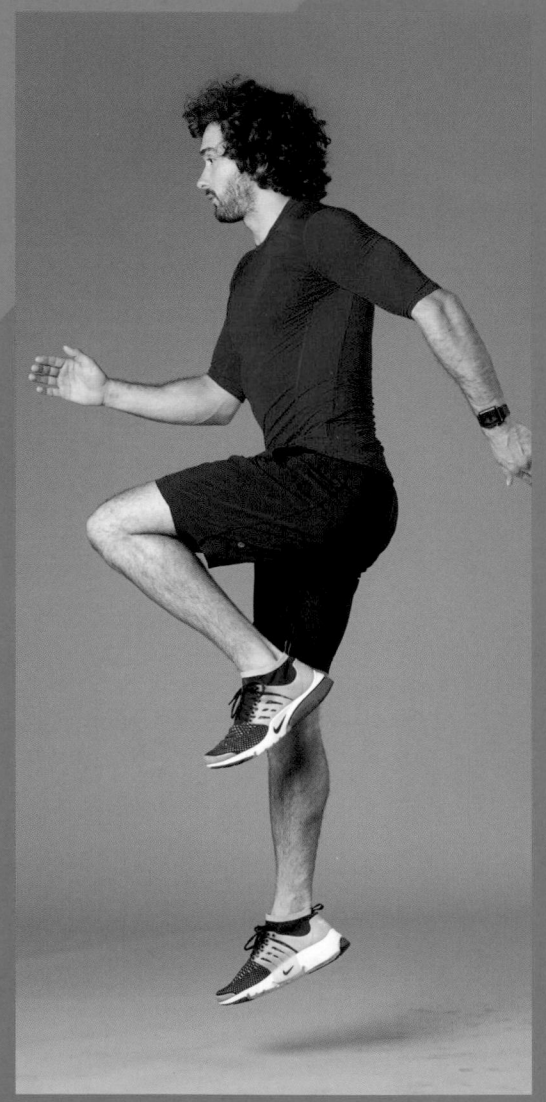

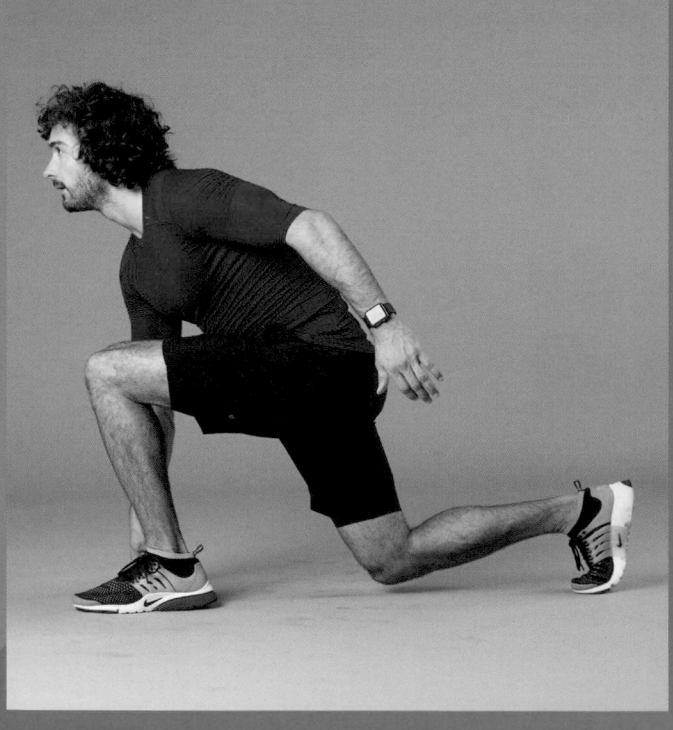

4. Glute bridges

Lie back on the floor and with one leg out straight out in front of you. With the other foot planted on the floor, drive your hips up off the ground by squeezing your hamstrings and glutes.

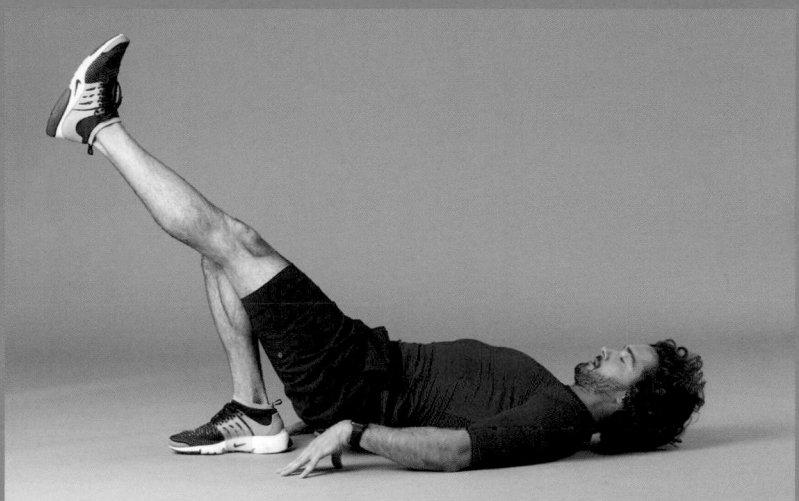

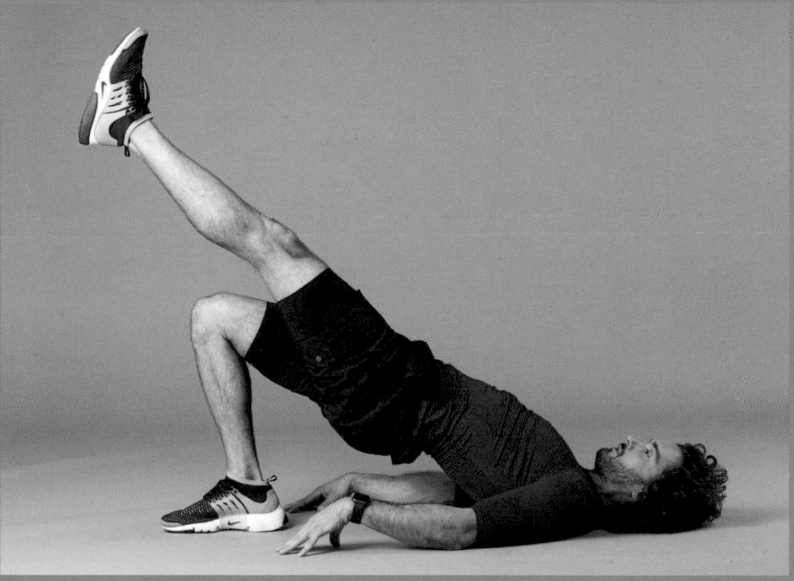

Beginner (3 rounds)	Intermediate (4 rounds)	Advanced (5 rounds)
20 seconds work	30 seconds work	40 seconds work
40 seconds rest	30 seconds rest	20 seconds rest

5. Squat pulses

Place your feet a comfortable distance apart and lower yourself as if you're about to sit into a chair. Rather than standing up fully, just pulse up and down staying low to keep the tension on your quads.

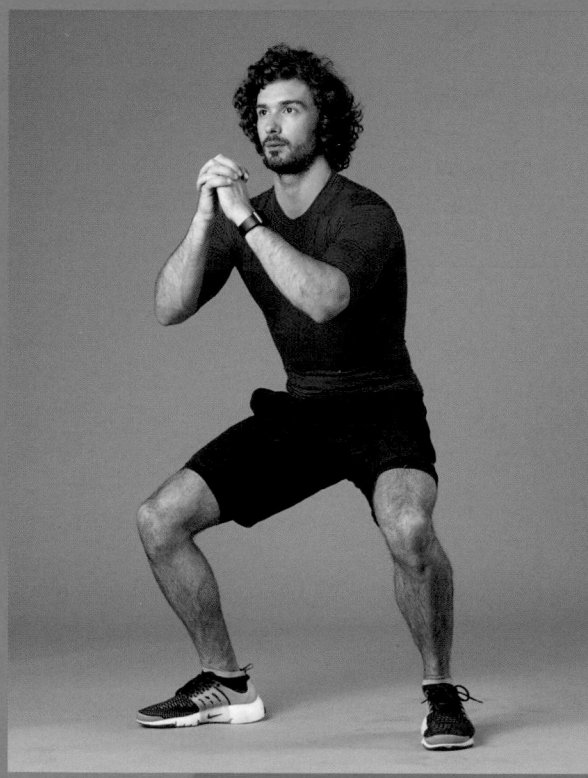
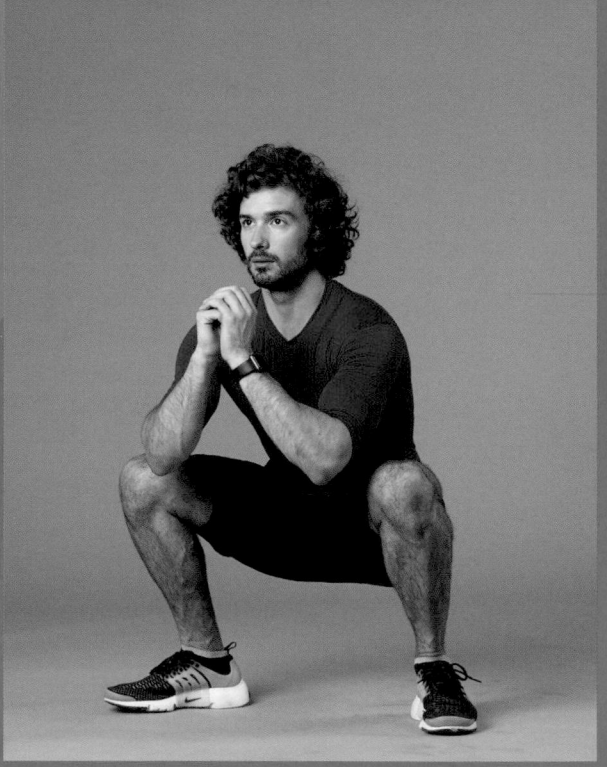

6. Walking plank

Start by holding yourself up in the push-up position and lower your body down one elbow at a time. Then push yourself up to the start position with one hand at a time. Repeat as many times as you can.

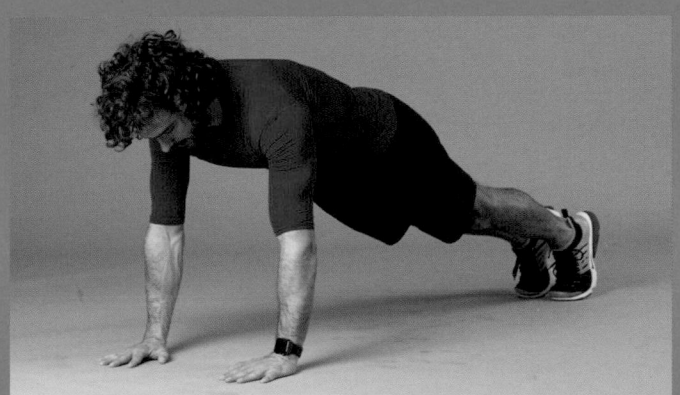

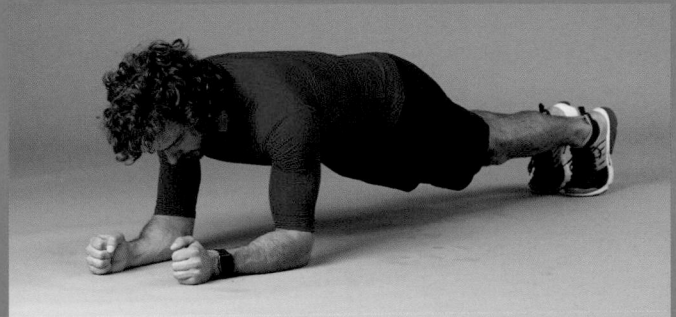

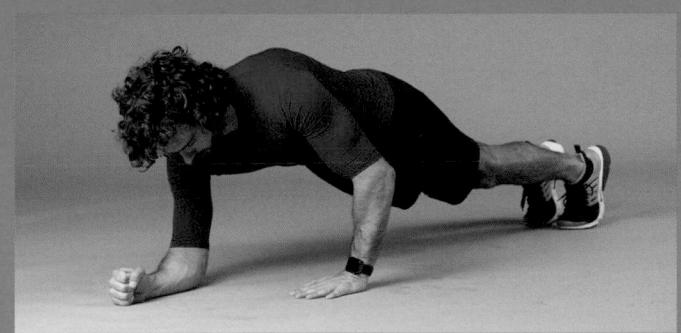

Beginner (3 rounds)	Intermediate (4 rounds)	Advanced (5 rounds)
20 seconds work	30 seconds work	40 seconds work
40 seconds rest	30 seconds rest	20 seconds rest

Weight-training Workout 1

I have included a beginner, intermediate and advanced level workout for the weight-training sessions with varying numbers of sets, reps and rest times. Each workout has 7 exercises in total to complete. If you are a beginner, for example, you will perform 10 reps on each exercise with a 60-second rest between each set. Do 3 sets on each exercise before moving on to the next one. As you progress to intermediate you will perform 4 sets of 12 reps with 45 seconds between each move.

TOP TIP

Invest in a set of adjustable dumbbells so you can easily change the resistance for different exercises based on your strength. Always aim to lift the weights with a slow and controlled tempo and try to increase your weights over time to make progress.

Don't be scared to lift heavy weights. More strength leads to greater lean muscle gains and that means you will increase your metabolism and burn more fat. If you are struggling on the final 2 reps of a set, then you know you have chosen the correct weight. If it feels too easy, you probably need to increase the weight.

1. Dumbbell squats

Choose a suitable weight. Hold one dumbbell in each arm and bend your knees to lower yourself into a squat position. Keep your back straight and chest up. Drive through the heels of your feet and clench your glutes at the top of the move.

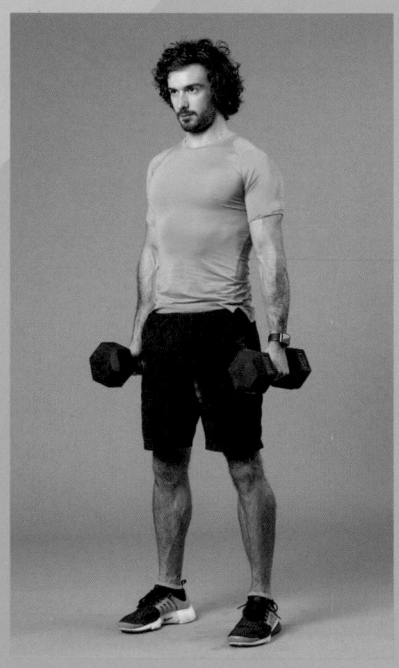
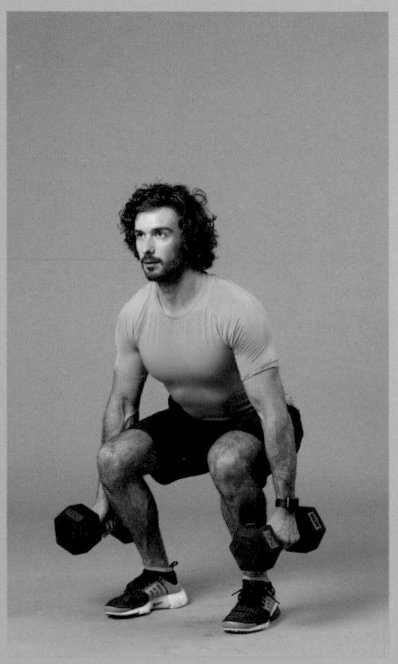

2. Shoulder press

Hold one dumbbell in each hand and lift them above your shoulders. Straighten your arms above your head and repeat.

You may find this exercise difficult to begin with, so be sure to select a suitable weight to start out. Once you master the movement pattern, aim to increase the weights.

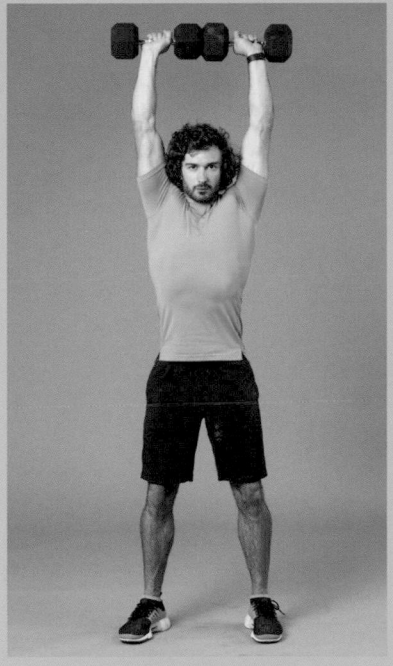
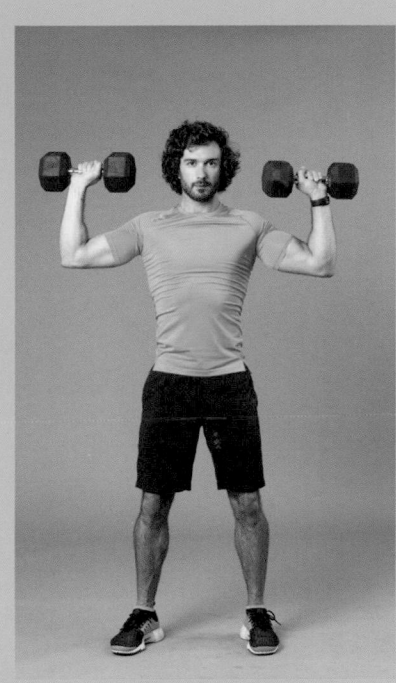

3. Reverse lunges

Lunges are my favourite lower-body exercise. Take a big step backwards, bending both knees and keeping your back straight. Drive up to a standing position and then alternate each leg.

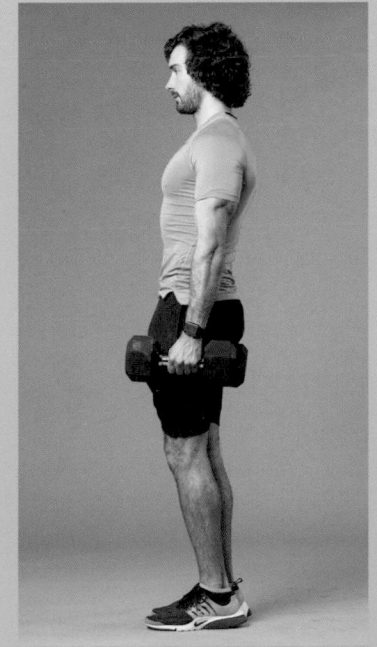
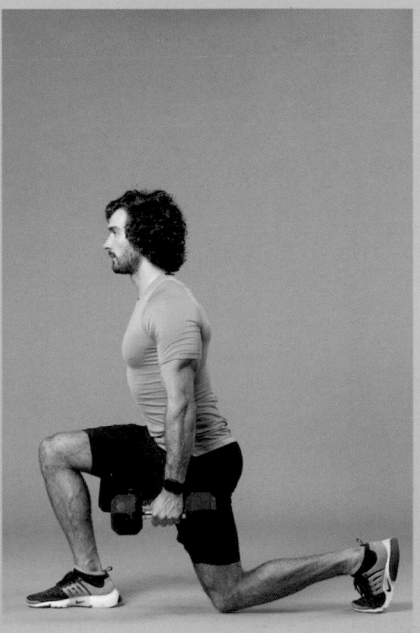

4. Chest press

Lower the dumbbells slowly towards your chest and press upwards bringing the weights together. If you don't have access to a bench you could also do this move on the floor.

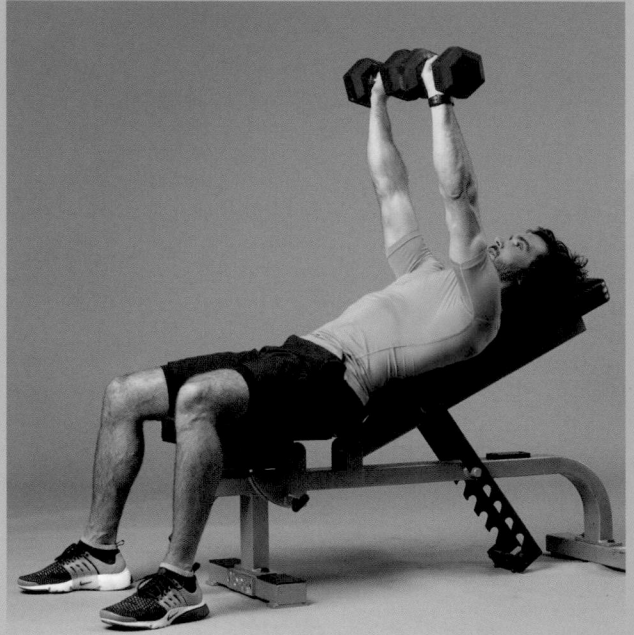

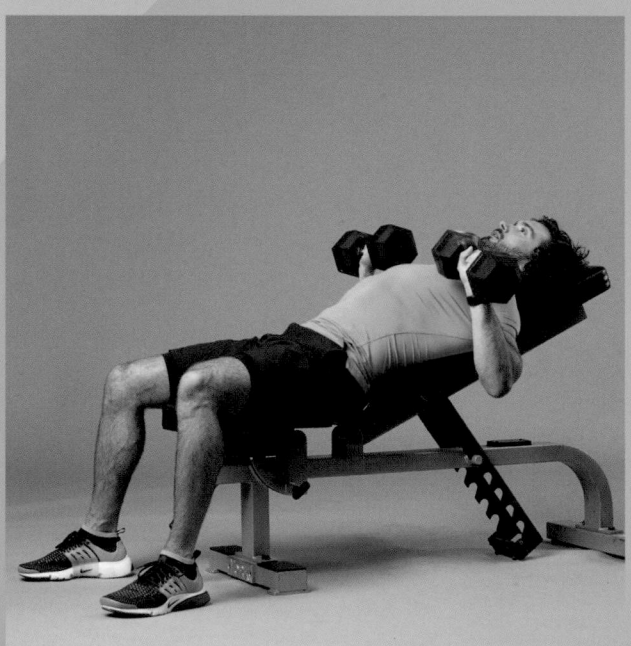

5. Single arm rows

Aim to keep the back flat and slowly lower the dumbbell towards the floor, then pull the dumbbell up towards the hip, keeping your body stable with no rotation.

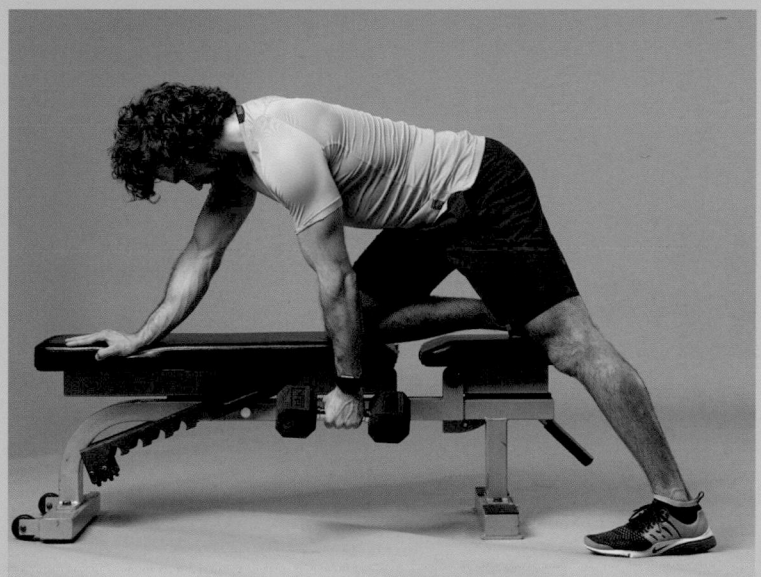

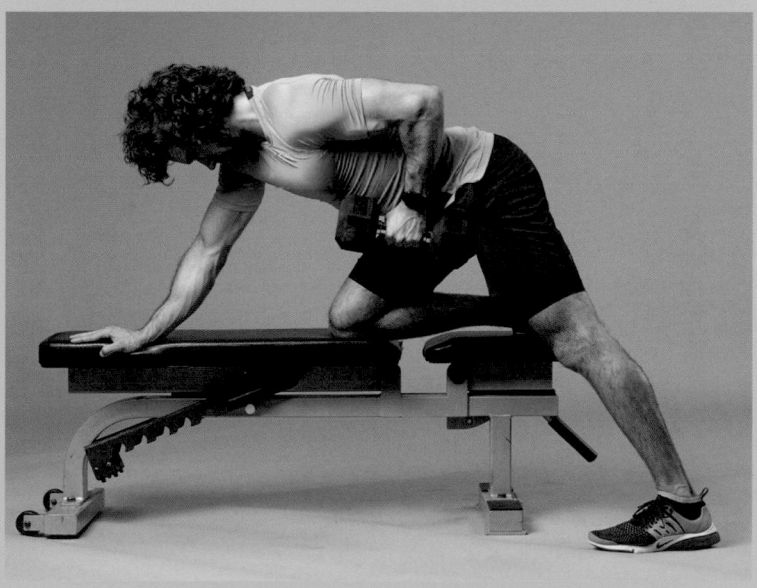

6. Bodyweight dips

This is a great exercise for working the bingo wings. Do the reps slow and controlled to really feel the burn. Keep your body close to the bench as you dip down and push up.

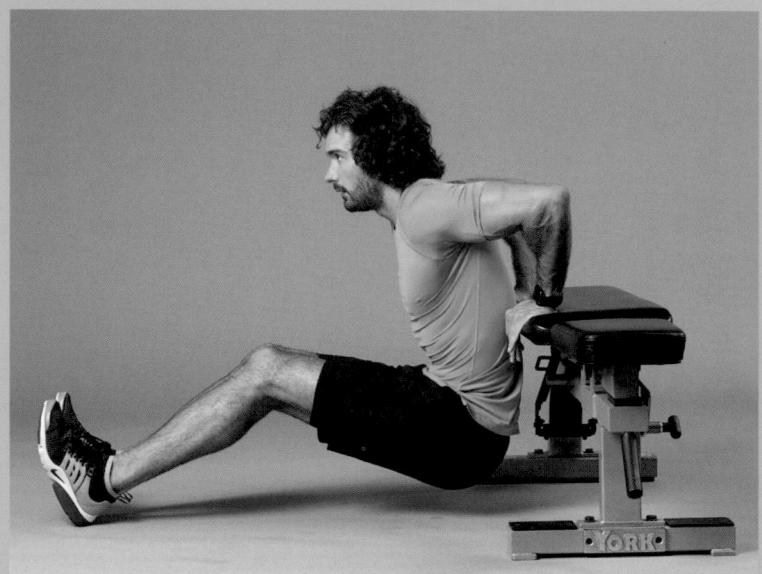

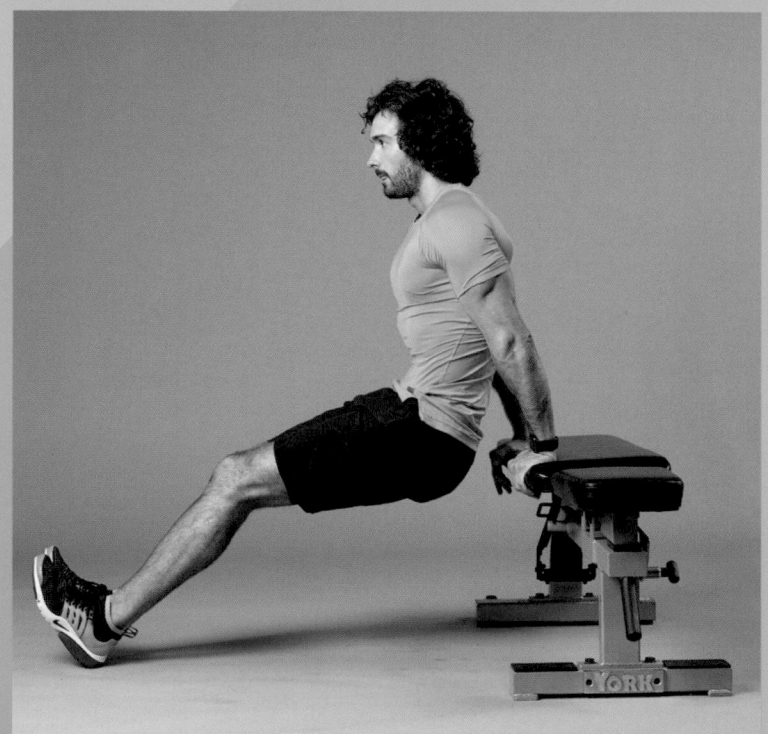

7. Reverse crunches

Lie flat and hold on to the bench
behind your head. Keep knees
bent and lower your legs away
from you, then pull your legs back
in towards you and drive your
hips off the bench using your abs.

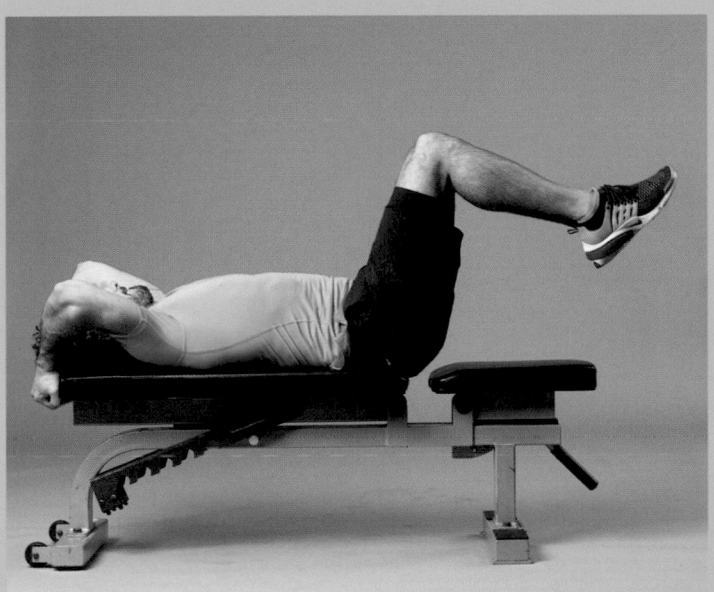
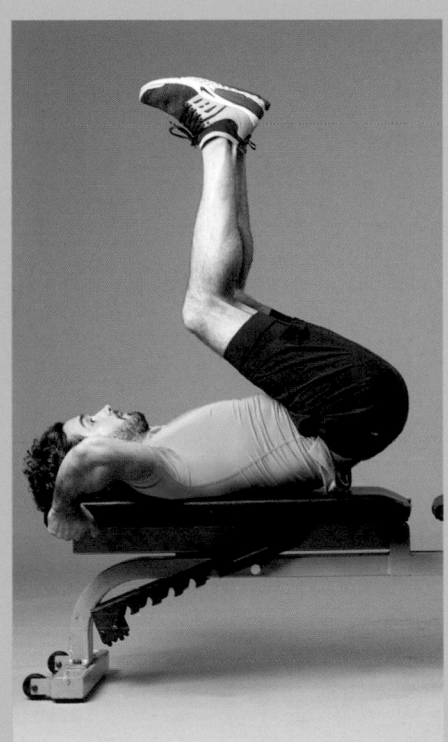

Beginner	Intermediate	Advanced
3 sets of 10 repeats	4 sets of 12 repeats	5 sets of 15 repeats
60 seconds rest	45 seconds rest	30 seconds rest

Weight-training Workout 2

1. Romanian dumbbell deadlifts

Keep your back straight, bend at the hips and lower the dumbbells towards the ground, keeping tension on the hamstrings. Stand up straight and repeat.

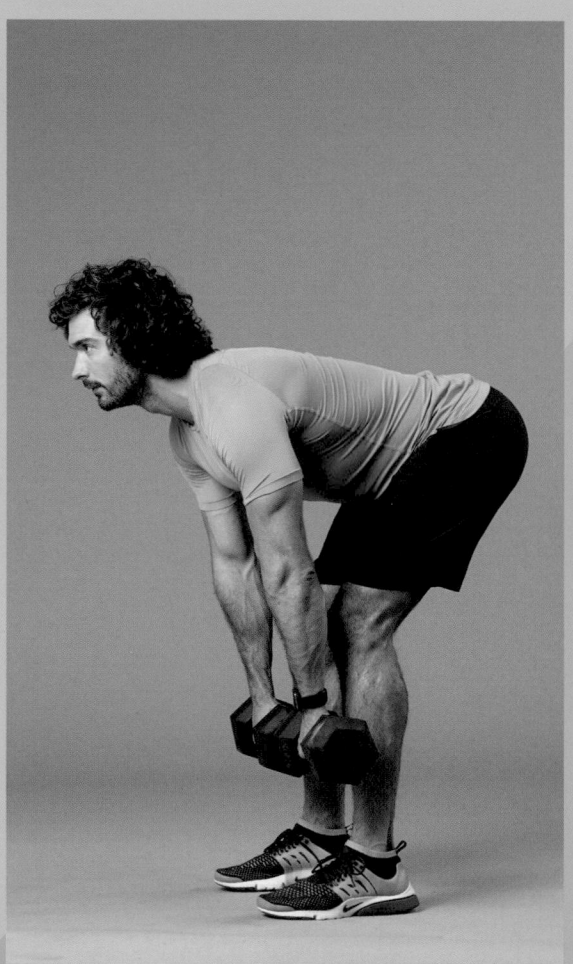
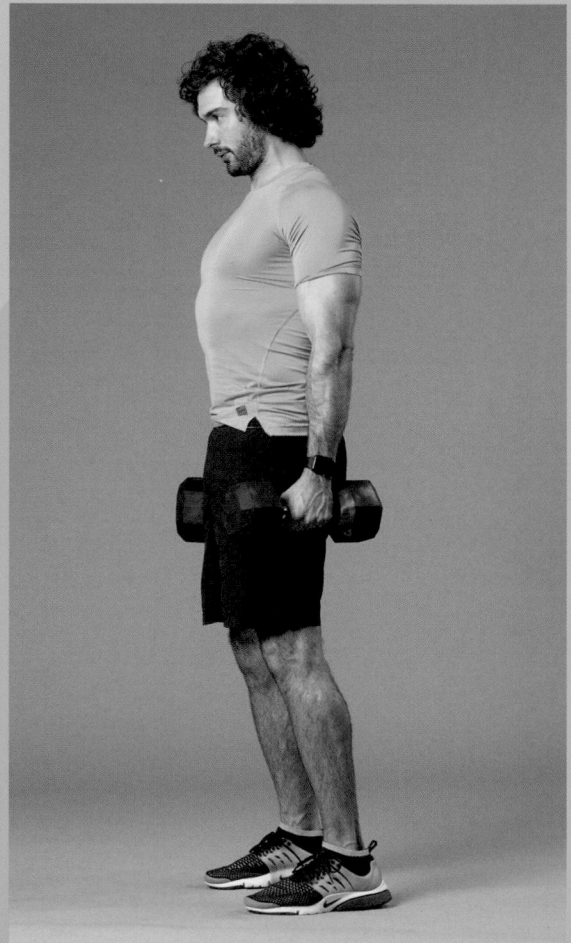

2. Box step-ups

Find a box, wall or bench to step on to. Hold one dumbbell in each arm and step up onto the box driving your knee up. Alternate between each leg.

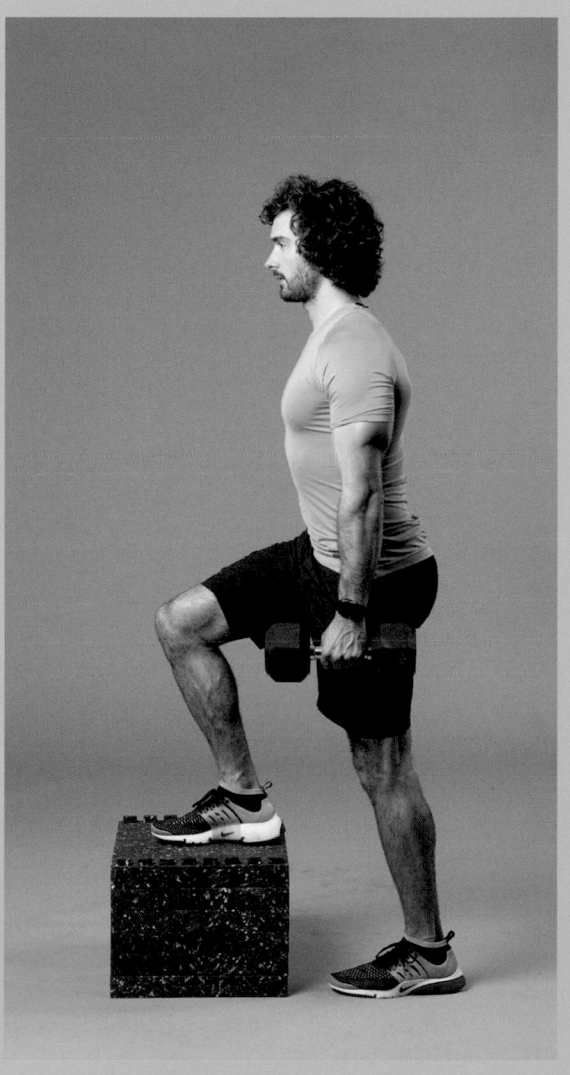
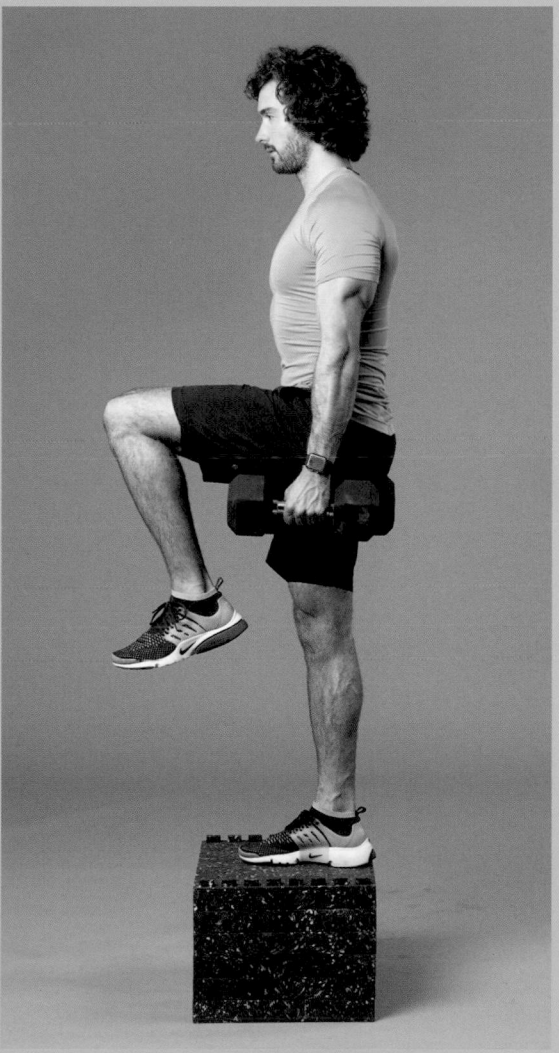

3. Bicep curls to shoulder press

This exercise combines two moves that target the biceps and your shoulders. First hammer curl the dumbbells and push straight up above the head.

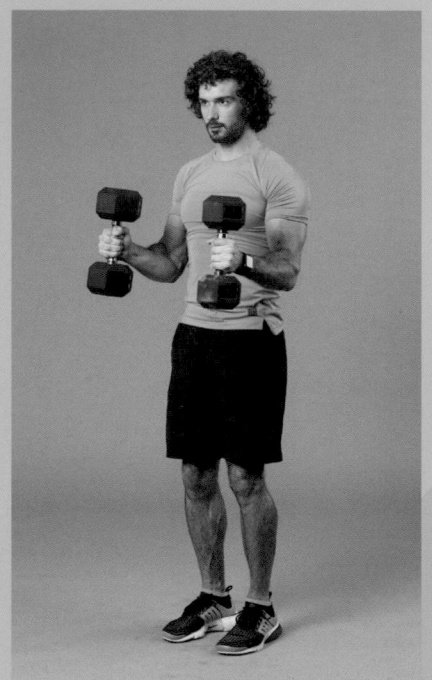

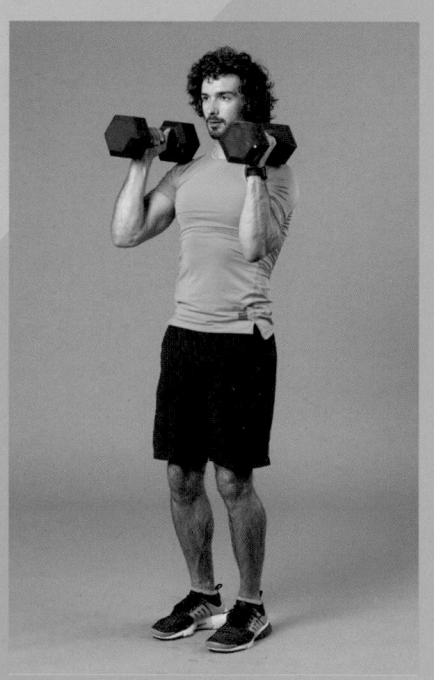

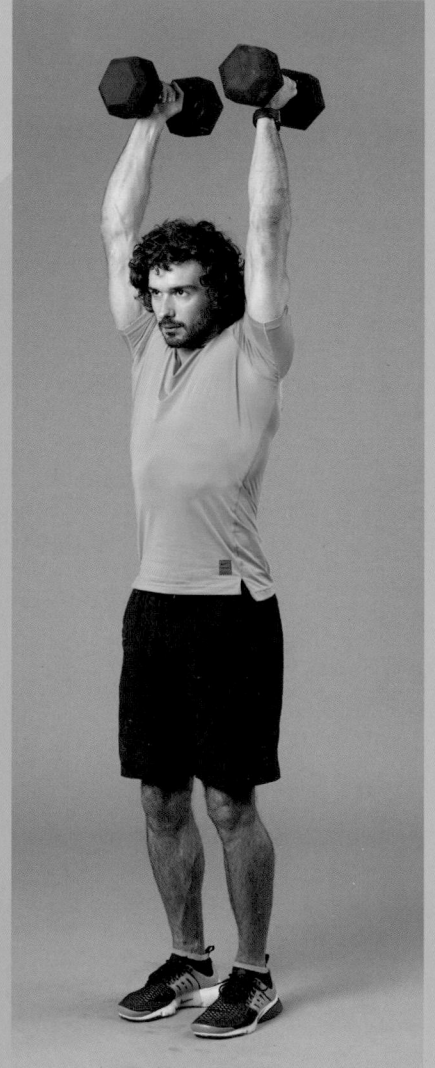

4. Tricep extensions

Stand up straight with one dumbbell in both hands. Slowly lower it behind you keeping your elbows close to your ears. Drive the dumbbell back up by extending your triceps.

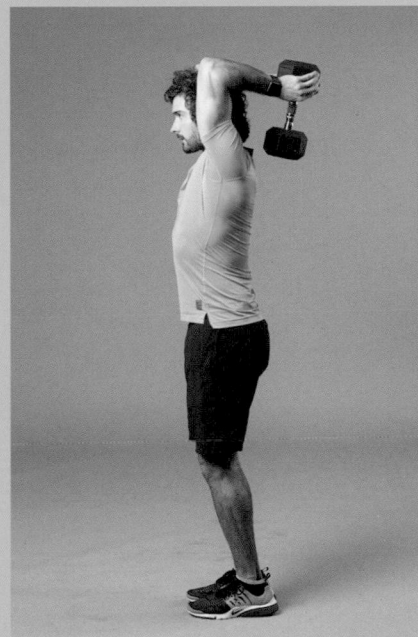
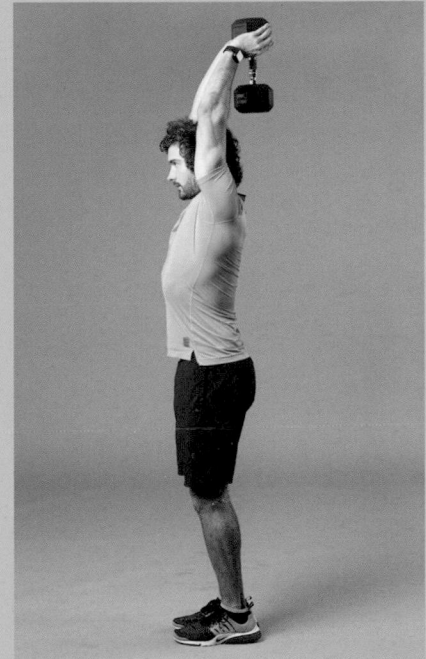

5. Wide sumo squats

Stand with your legs wide and feet turned out like a sumo wrestler. Holding one dumbbell close to your chest, slowly lower yourself towards the ground and then stand up, driving through the heels of your feet.

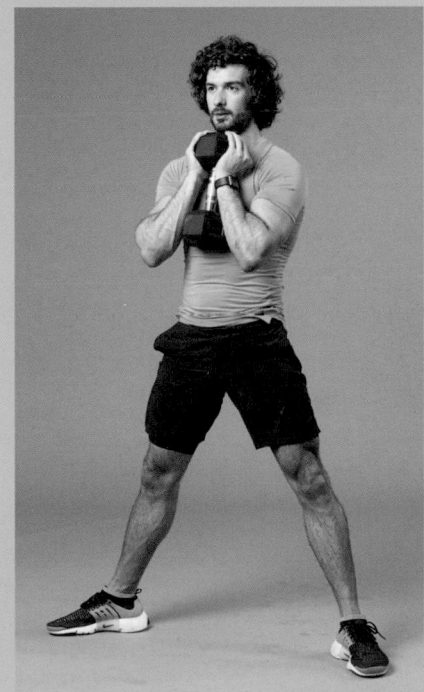
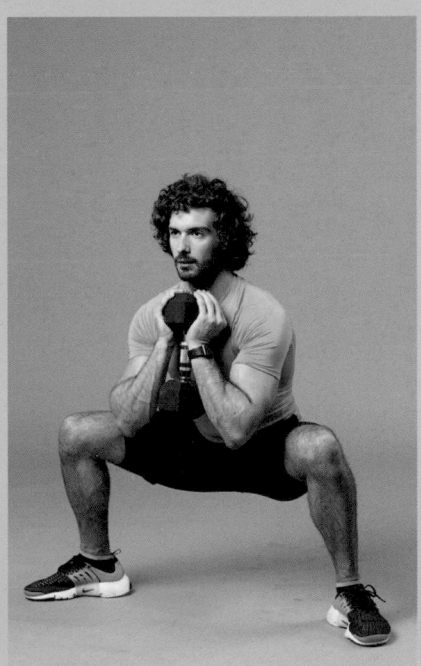

6. Lateral raises

Hold one dumbbell in each hand and, using your shoulders, raise them up each side until they are parallel with the ground. Repeat this move, keeping slow and controlled.

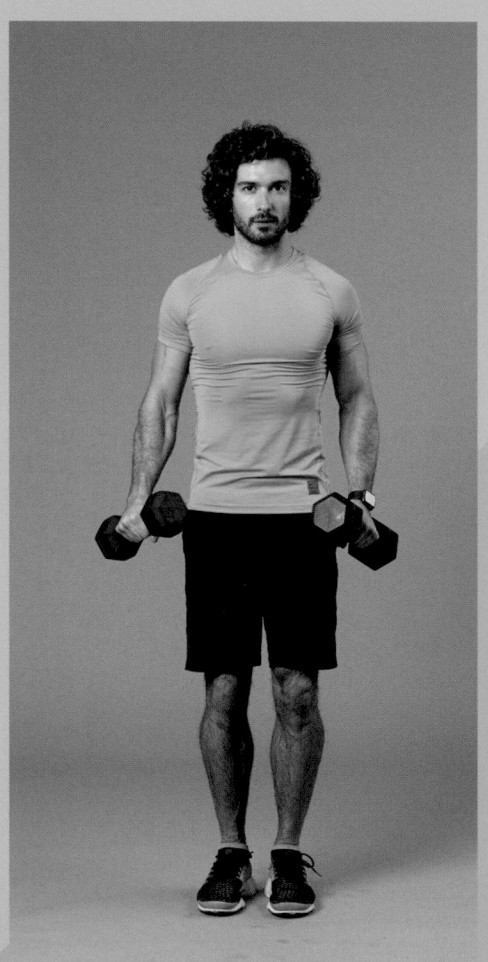
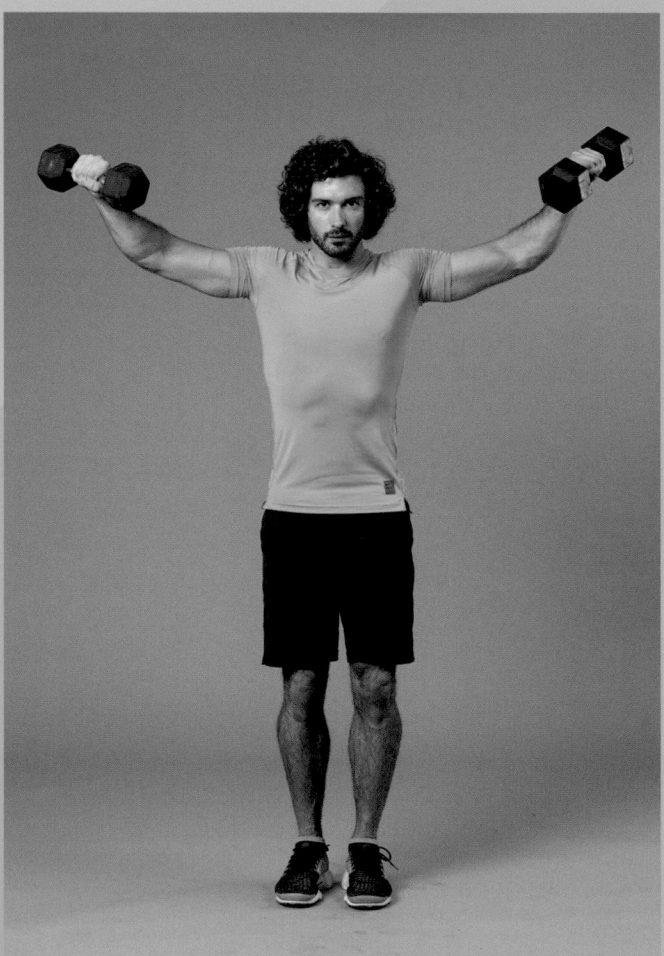

7. Sit-ups

If you are a beginner to sit-ups then just do this exercise without the weight. When you feel ready to progress, simply hold a light weight close to your chest to add resistance to the move.

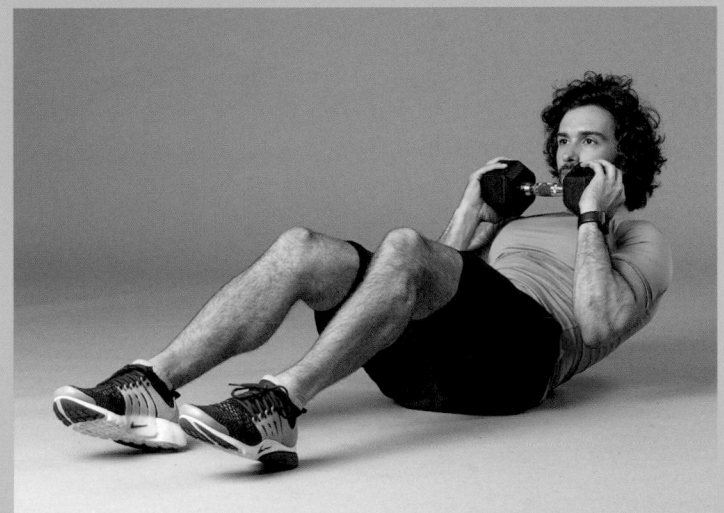

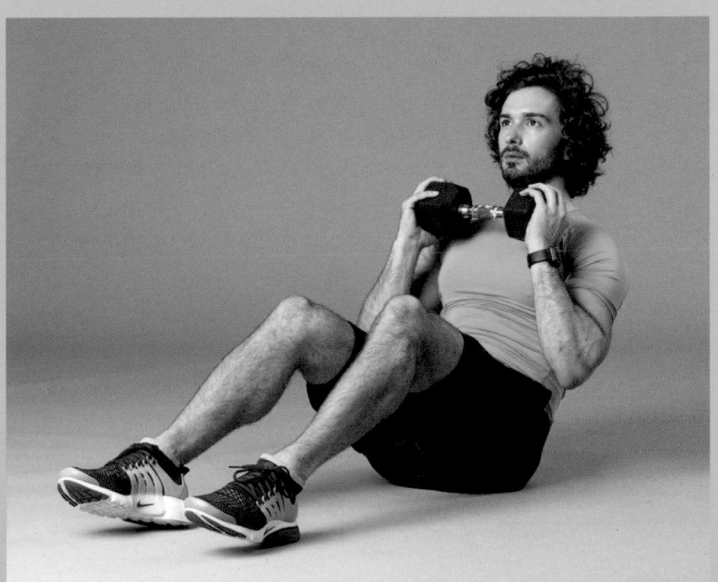

Beginner	Intermediate	Advanced
3 sets of 10 repeats	4 sets of 12 repeats	5 sets of 15 repeats
60 seconds rest	45 seconds rest	30 seconds rest

HIIT machine cardio

You may be someone who prefers to do HIIT on cardio machines as opposed to using your own body weight. This is perfectly fine, just try to challenge yourself every now and again by using a variety of equipment. My personal favourites are treadmill and bike sprints, so I switch between the two. The emphasis on HIIT is to really push as hard as possible on the working set. If you are a beginner, you will be working to your max effort for 20 seconds followed by 40 seconds rest. You will repeat this for a total of 15 minutes for beginner, 20 minutes for intermediate and 25 minutes for advanced. Train hard, stay focused and watch your fitness go through the roof and your body fat melt away.

You can apply HIIT training to any of the below pieces of equipment.

Treadmill sprints

These are my favourite HIIT. Run as fast as you can, then either reduce the speed and walk for your rest period, or come to a complete stop. To really make this a challenge, try increasing the incline or simply do it outdoors by doing hill sprints.

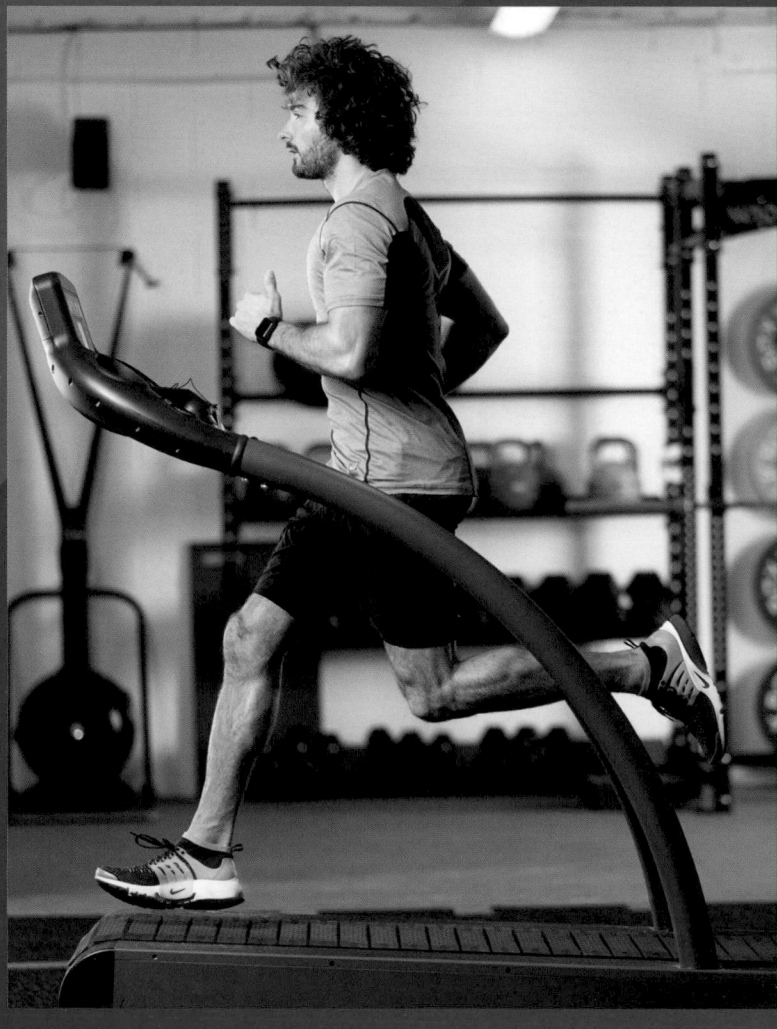

Bike

This is a much lower-impact form of cardio, so it's ideal for people who don't enjoy running or have issues with their knees. Crank up the resistance and pedal as hard and fast as you can, then reduce the resistance to near zero to let your legs recover before attacking the next sprint interval.

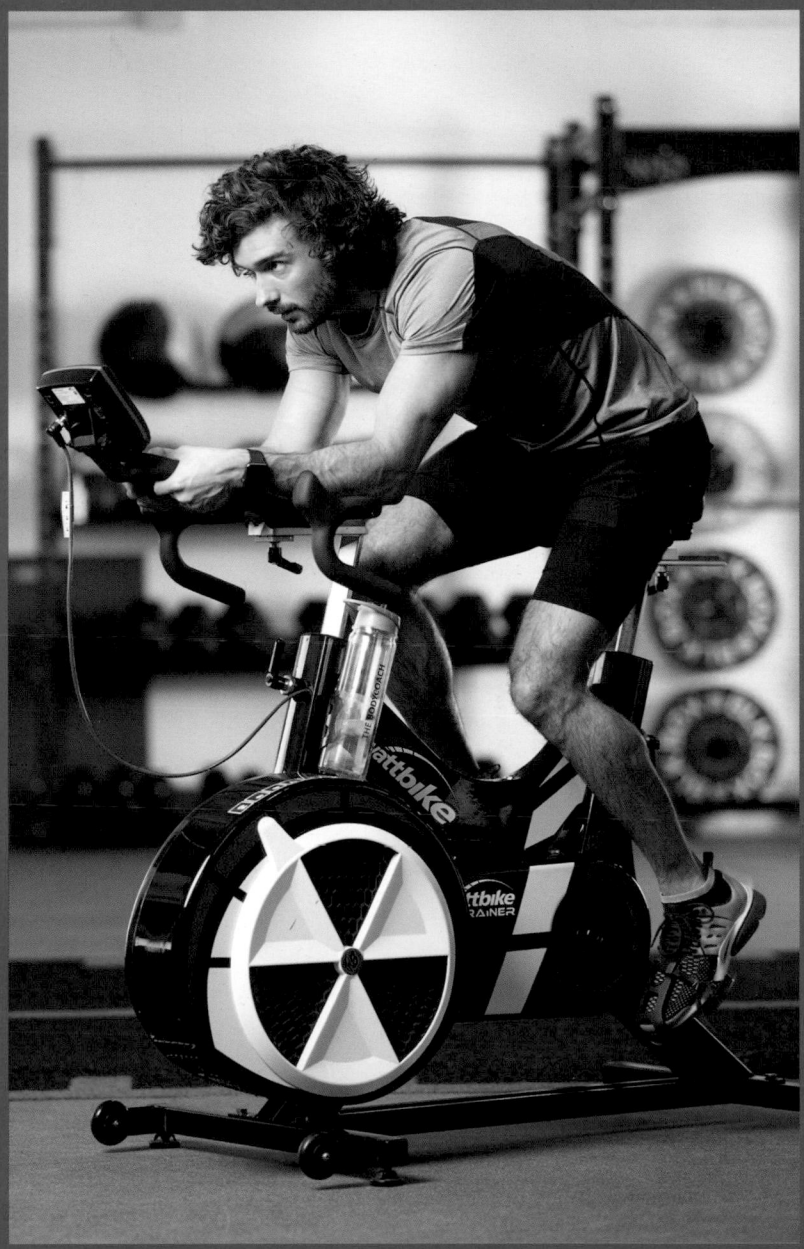

HIIT machine cardio

Rower

This exercise is a full-body workout and will really get your lungs working. It uses lots of muscle groups, including your back, arms and legs, so it's going to be intense. Row as hard as possible with a heavy resistance then reduce the resistance and come to a slow recovery pace before sprinting all-out again.

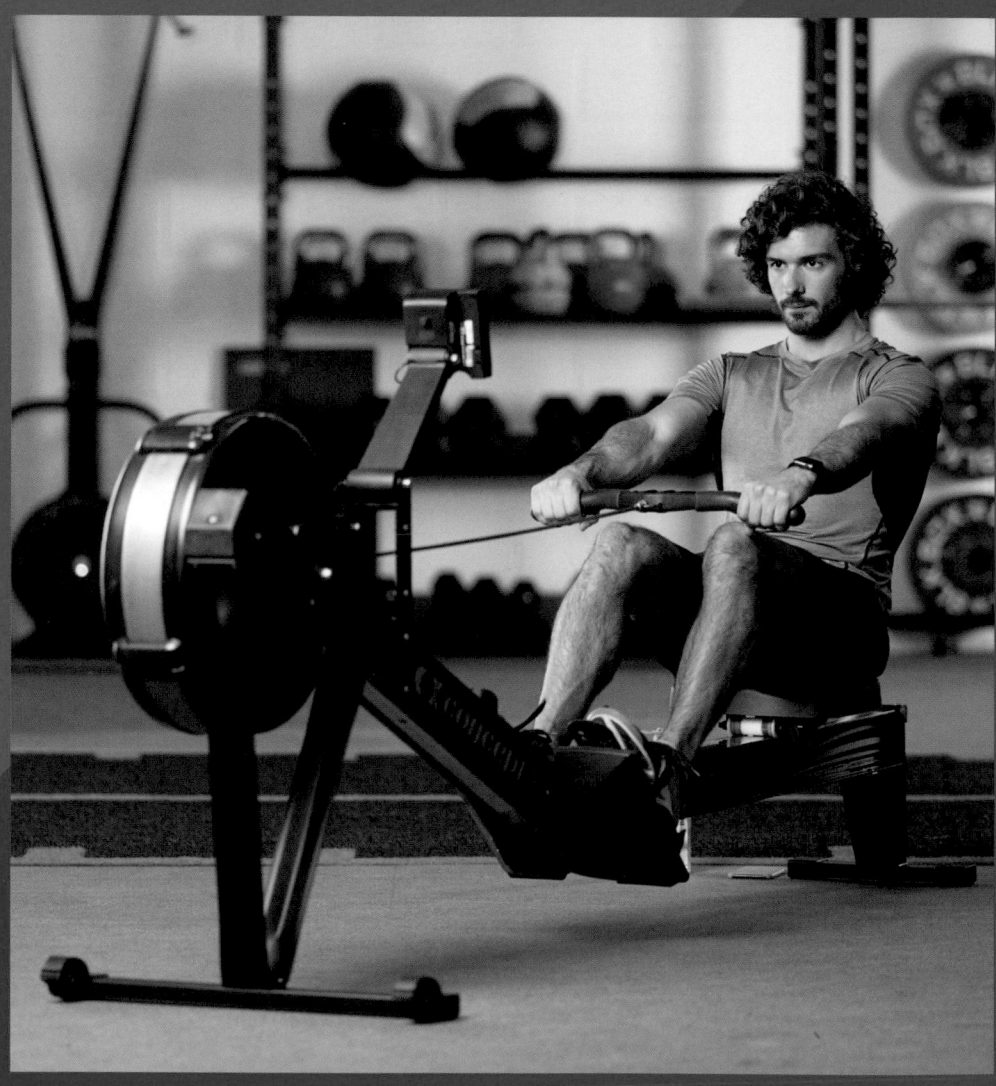

Assault bike

In my opinion this is the most brutal and challenging piece of cardio equipment on earth. It combines a cross-trainer with a bike and the result is a gut-busting combination that makes your whole body work extremely hard. Same as the bike, just go hard for a short burst, recover, suck as much air in your lungs and repeat. Good luck!

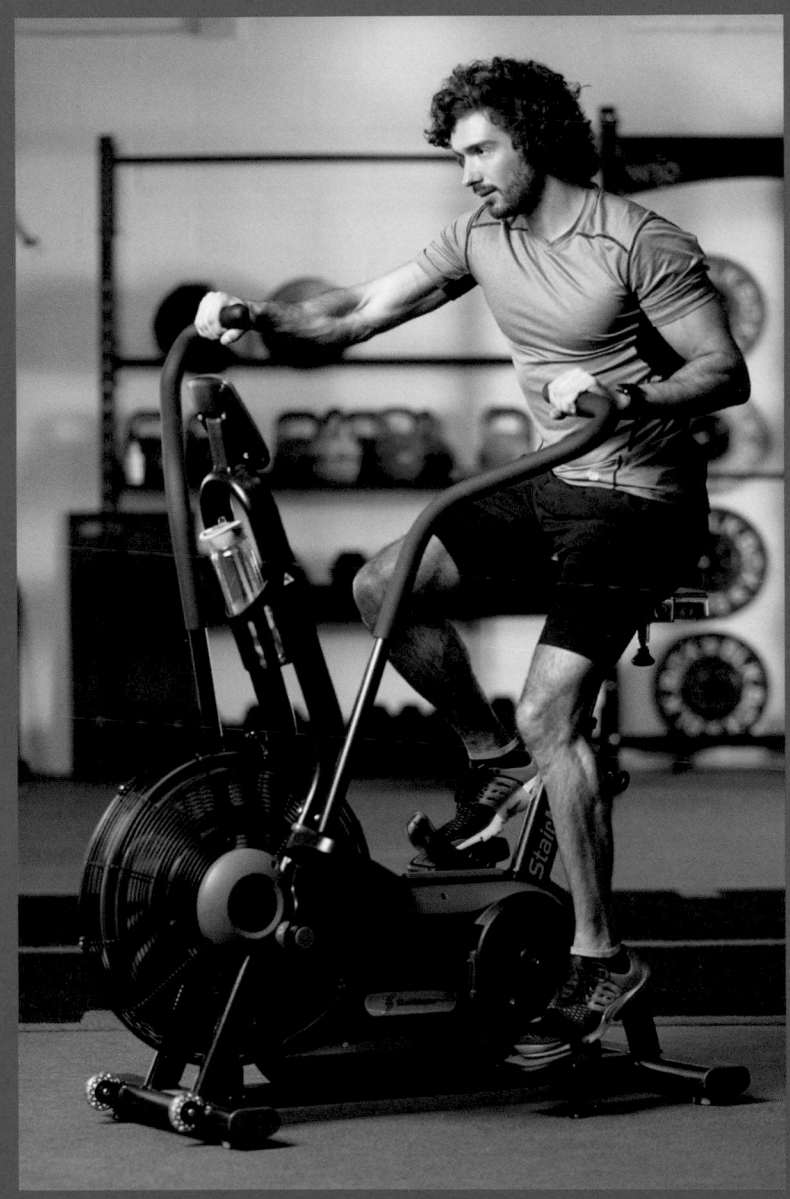

HIIT machine cardio

Battle ropes

The battle ropes are great pieces of equipment that you can purchase and use at home if you don't have access to any cardio machines. Holding one end of the rope in each hand, wave the ropes up and down as high and fast as you can. Then drop the ropes, rest, recover and repeat.

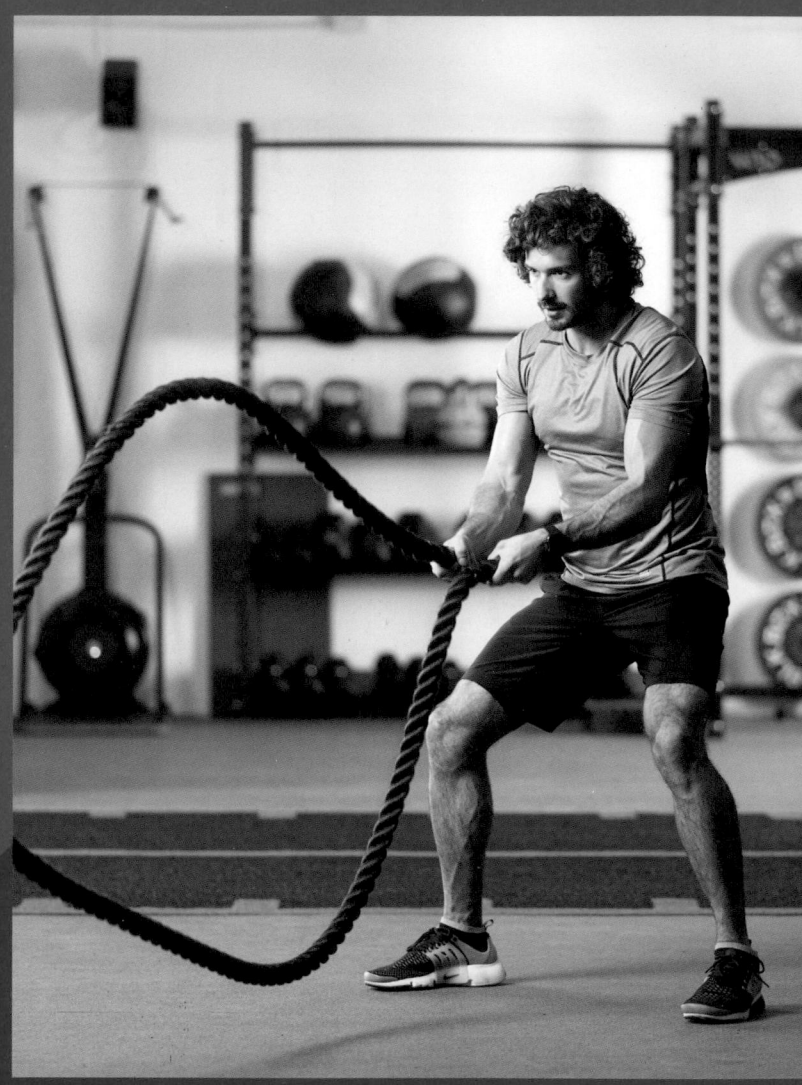

Beginner (15 mins)	Intermediate (20 mins)	Advanced (25 mins)
20 seconds work	30 seconds work	40 seconds work
40 seconds rest	30 seconds rest	20 seconds rest

Cool down

HIIT training is very intense; usually the last thing you want to do afterwards is sit down and stretch, but it really is essential if you want to get the most out of this plan. I used to neglect my stretching as I had no discipline with it, but all it did was leave me with unnecessary injuries. I've got better now, though, because I'm in the routine of stretching at the end of each session for at least 5–10 minutes.

I recommend doing a 5-minute dynamic warm-up before each session and then holding static stretches afterwards. Try to always stretch all the major muscles, including the hamstrings, quads and hip flexors. Aim to hold each stretch for 30 seconds before moving on to the next. Another great thing to do for recovery is foam rolling. You can buy these online really cheap or most gyms have them in the stretching areas now, so give that a go, too.

By stretching and foam rolling you will reduce the risk of injury, become more mobile and recover quicker. This means you can be ready to smash your next workout and really get the most out of each session.

Good luck with *The Fat-Loss Plan*. Believe in yourself, take action and be consistent. The results will come.

Index

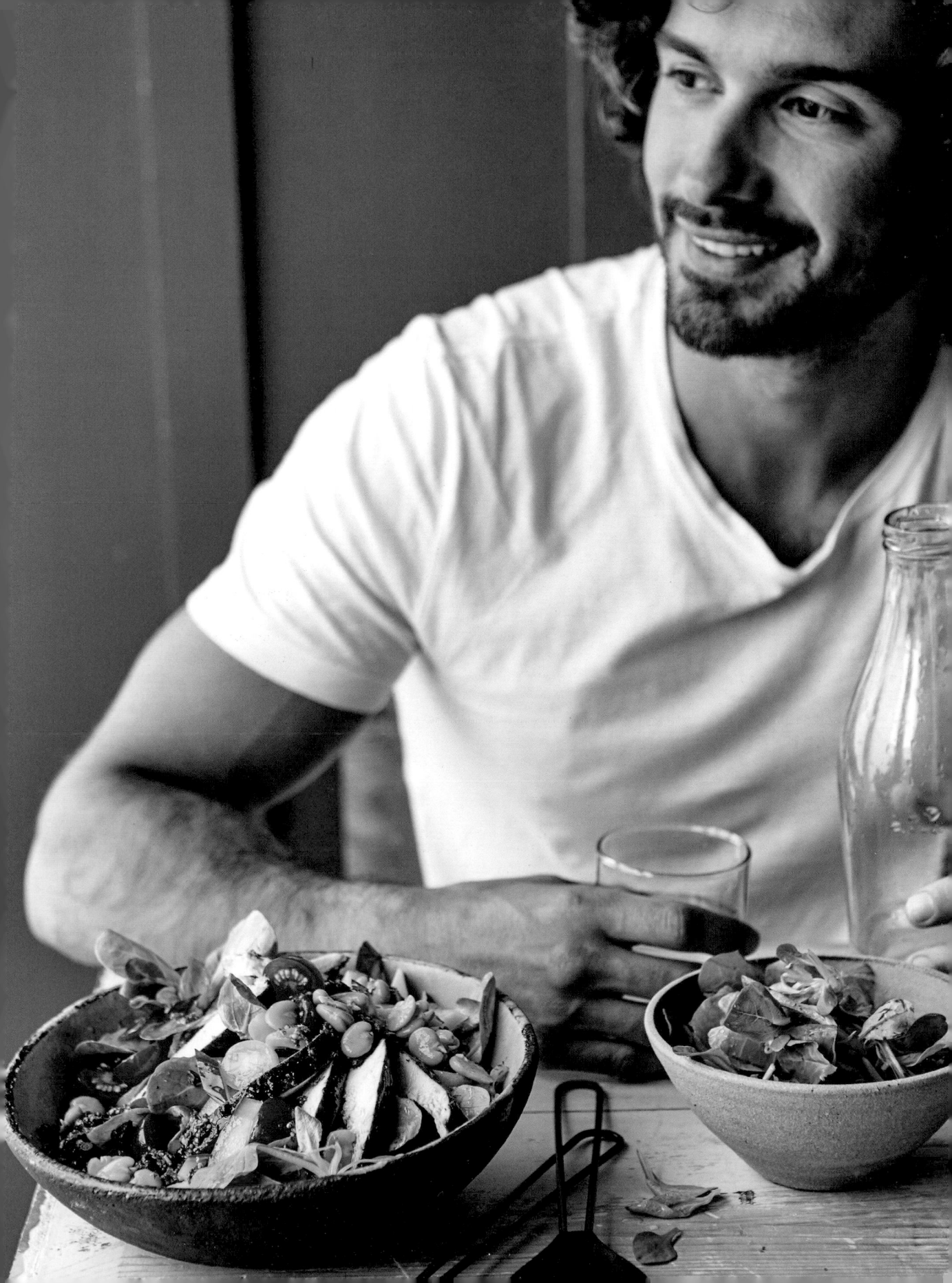

Thank yous

I would like to say a big thank you firstly to Carole, Martha, Hockley, Maja and Bianca for helping me create such a wonderful cookbook. I'm really proud of this one and I feel very lucky to have you on my team. To my family, my friends and my sidekick: I love you all.

THE **BODYCOACH**

The Body Coach 90 Day Plan

Join the hundreds of thousands of people around the world that have transformed their body with my tailored 90 day meal and exercise plans. To sign up go to **www.thebodycoach.com**